Gail Rae-Garwood

SlowItDownCKD

2022

Gail Rae-Garwood

Gail Rae-Garwood

SlowItDownCKD 2022

Copyright © 2022 Gail Rae-Garwood

All rights reserved.

Gail Rae-Garwood

Dedication

All the books in the **SlowItDownCKD** series are dedicated to my readers:

those that asked questions,

those that didn't,

and those that wish they had.

Here's hoping all the answers you seek are in these **SlowItDownCKD** blogs from 2022.

Gail Rae-Garwood

Introduction

When my family doctor told me fifteen years ago that I probably had a problem with my kidneys, my first reaction was to demand in no uncertain terms, "What is it and how did I get it?" Hence, the title of my first chronic kidney disease (CKD) book. There are many, many of us out there. By us, I mean those who have CKD, although friends and family of CKD patients can also gain insight into the daily life of those of us living with the disease via this collection of 2022's **SlowItDownCKD** blogs.

This is not an improvement over the earlier books in the **SlowItDownCKD** series, but – rather - an addition which covers topics I hadn't thought of in previous years or those that readers asked about last year. I am no expert, but I did want to know what was happening to me on a daily basis and what new discoveries there were that might help slow down this deterioration of my kidney function. Apparently, so do my readers.

The more you know about chronic kidney disease, the more comfortable you'll feel. I sure wish someone had blogged about it when it was new to me. I've discovered my readers are eager to tell me what they want to know about. I research for them and respond with a blog post but remind them they need to speak with their medical team first and foremost. And I repeatedly remind them I am not a doctor.

I've written other books about chronic kidney disease that you may find referenced in the blogs. These are *What Is It and How Did I Get It? Early Stage Chronic Kidney Disease, SlowItDownCKD 2011, SlowItDownCKD 2012, SlowItDownCKD 2013, SlowItDownCKD 2014, SlowItDownCKD 2015, SlowItDownCKD 2016, SlowItDownCKD 2017, SlowItDownCKD 2018, SlowItDownCKD 2019, SlowItDownCKD 2020,* and *SlowItDownCKD 2021.*

In the interest of keeping this book from becoming mammoth, I've deleted the pictures, diagrams, and news of past events. I also removed my signature closing, "Until next week, keep living your life!" After all, how many times can you read the same sentence in a single book?

Welcome to *SlowItDownCKD 2022.*

Gail Rae-Garwood

Topics by Date

1/3   Basics

1/10 Covid Safety

1/17 Born with Kidney Disease

1/24 Insulin

1/31 Skin

2/7   Street Drugs

2/14 Jail and Prison Inmates

2/21 Black Nephrologists

2/28 Undocumented Immigrants

3/7   Kidney Stories Toastmasters Club

3/14 Phosphorous, Protein, Potassium, and Sodium

3/21 More Dialysate Needed

3/28 Acute Tubular Necrosis (ATN)

4/4   Fluids

4/11 Water Apps

4/18 Holiday Meal Leftovers

4/25 Renal Support Network (RSN)

5/2   Kidney Disease Cookbooks

5/9   My Kidney Disease Advocacy

5/16 Pets

5/23 Lead in the Water

6/6   Low Blood Sugar

6/13 Pancreas/Kidney Transplant

6/20 Weight Loss Insulin

6/27 Potassium and Phosphorous in the Different Kidney Diets

7/4   Protein in the Different Kidney Diets

7/11 Sodium/Salt in the Different Kidney Diets

7/18 Supplanting Dialysis

7/25 Your Nails

8/1   The Pancreas

8/8   Super Taster

8/15 Exercise

8/22 Dried Urine Test for Comprehensive Hormones (DUTCH)e

8/29 Continuous Glucose Monitoring (CGM) Devices

9/5   Pizza

SlowItDownCKD 2022

9/12   Hydroxymethylbutyrate (HMB)

9/19   American Association of Kidney Patients (AAKP)

9/26   Patient-Centered Outcomes Research Institute (PCORI)

10/3   Atypical Hemolytic Uremic Syndrome (aHus)

10/10 National Organization for Rare Disorders (NORD)l

10/17 New eGFR calculations for Blacks

10/24 The Asian Kidney Disease Equation/James Meyer's Face book Groups

10/31 Pediatric Urine Reflux

11/7   Online and In Person Support Groups

11/14 Seasonal Effects on eGFR

11/21 Pediatric Vesicoureteral Reflux Again

11/28 Horseshoe Kidney [Renal Fusion]

12/5   Edema

12/12 Kidney Development

12/19 Duplex Kidneys

12/26 Pneumonia & CKD

SlowItDownCKD 2022

Gail Rae-Garwood

1/3 **What Are the Basics, Anyway?**

Happy New Year! You know, the only way for it to be happy is for you to make it happy. For us, that includes taking care of our chronic kidney disease in the most basic ways. "Remind me; what are those?" my good buddy asked when I said that to her. So, this will be a back-to-basics blog to begin the new year.

We all know that what we eat has a lot of influence on our kidneys. Way back when I was writing **What Is It and How Did I Get It? Early Stage Chronic Kidney Disease**, I called this influence "the three p's and an s." That's an easy way to remember what I'll explain next. Remember though, we are each unique patients and you and your nephrologist will decide to what extent you follow these suggestions.

Okay then. Let's start. MedlinePlus has a comprehensive explanation of potassium:

"Potassium is a mineral that your body needs to work properly. It is a type of electrolyte. It helps your nerves to function and muscles to contract. It helps your heartbeat stay regular. It also helps move nutrients into cells and waste products out of cells. A diet rich in potassium helps to offset some of sodium's harmful effects on blood pressure....

Your kidneys help to keep the right amount of potassium in your body. If you have chronic kidney disease, your kidneys may not remove extra potassium from the blood.... You may need a special diet to lower the amount of potassium that you eat."

Then there's protein. We're pretty familiar with the definition, but what does it has to do with your kidneys? The National Kidney Foundation has that one covered:

".... Protein is used to build muscle, heal, fight infection, and stay healthy. Protein needs vary based on your age, sex and overall general health. Protein in the diet comes from both animal and plant sources....

You need protein every day to meet your body's needs, but if you have kidney disease, your body may not be able to remove all the waste from the protein in your diet. Excess protein waste can build up in your blood causing nausea, loss of appetite, weakness, and taste changes....

The more protein waste that needs to be removed, the harder the kidneys need to work to get rid of it. This can be stressful for your kidneys, causing them to wear out faster. For people with kidney disease who are not on dialysis, a diet lower in protein is recommended."

The final 'p' is phosphorous. I turned to WebMD for help with this one:

"Phosphorus is a mineral, likeiron [sic] or potassium. You have more of this mineral in your body than any other except calcium....

It plays an important role in keeping you healthy, so it's an important part of your diet. One of its main tasks is to serve as a building block for healthy teeth and bones. You may think that's calcium's job. But calcium needs phosphorus to make your teeth and bones strong.

Phosphorus also helps your nerves and muscles do their jobs. It's a buffer that keeps the pH level in your blood balanced. Phosphorus also helps you turn fat, carbs, and protein into energy....

When they work well, your kidneys remove extra phosphorus your body can't use.

If you have a kidney condition like chronic kidney disease, you may have high levels of phosphorus. This can cause your bones to lose calcium or calcium deposits to form in your blood vessels, eyes, heart, and lungs. If you have too much phosphorus in your body for a long period of time, your chance of a heart attack or stroke goes up."

Wow, and we're not done yet. There's sodium, too. The to the MayoClinic for the following:

"The body needs some sodium to function properly. Sodium plays a role in:

The balance of fluids in your body

The way nerves and muscles work

The kidneys balance the amount of sodium in the body. When sodium is low, the kidneys hold on to it. When sodium is high, the kidneys release some in urine.

If the kidneys can't eliminate enough sodium, it builds up in the blood. Sodium attracts and holds water, so the blood volume increases. The heart must work harder to pump blood, and that increases pressure in the arteries. Over time this can increase the risk of heart disease, stroke and kidney disease.

Some people are more sensitive to the effects of sodium than are others. That means they retain sodium more easily, which leads to fluid retention and increased blood pressure."

Now you can understand the plethora of kidney diet cookbooks. Or you can limit these electrolytes yourself. That's what I did until I developed diabetes. I've had CKD for 14 years, so some of the estimating had become rote. Honestly, now I'm back to needing help to combine the renal and diabetes diet.

Dealing with "the three p's and one s" is the *beginning* of taking care of your CKD. There's also exercise, sleep, avoiding stress, rest, watching your weight, avoiding alcohol, and smoking, and keeping tight control of your diabetes, heart disease, and high blood pressure. Oh, limiting your sodium will help you with your high blood pressure, too.

There isn't enough space in this particular blog to write about each of those. Let me know if you'd like a blog explaining more about the items in the previous paragraph. Meanwhile, see what you [or you and doctor] can do to help with them.

Welcome to 2022, the year you take a bigger part in making yourself happy by taking care of your CKD.

1/10 *We Interrupt...*

Wow, just wow. I had intended to keep writing about the basics of chronic kidney disease today, but I just spoke with my nephrologist via FaceTime. That's a call I had waited over a month to have, even though my GFR had dropped 20 points. I thought the drop constituted the need for an immediate callback from him, but he just didn't have the time. He was overwhelmed with the hospitalized Covid patients who needed dialysis.

During our talk today, he told me it isn't just nephrology that's affected. All specialties are now three months out for appointments. Three months! There's a shortage of staff due to Covid, including doctors that specialize in a specific organ.

I found this downright scary until he explained that this variant, Omicron, probably will not spike as long as the others have. At least that's the latest prognosis. I did find that comforting. My GFR has resumed its usual number, so I can afford to be comforted by this. I think of others who have immediate medical problems and I cringe.

How, in heaven's name, can we improve this situation? How can we help? First and foremost, get your vaccine. My husband and I are fortunate enough to have had both Moderna vaccines and the Moderna booster with nothing more than a sore arm for a day or two as a side effect. I know not everyone is that lucky. I also know it's worth whatever side-effects you have. My grown children lost their father to Covid before there were vaccines available.

Are the vaccines safe for us? I'll let the National Kidney Foundation answer that question:

"While the effectiveness rates of COVID-19 vaccines are very good, we now know that people who are on immunosuppression medications for the treatment of advanced kidney disease and kidney transplant recipients, may not receive the same level of protection, also known as antibody immunity, from the COVID-19 vaccine as people who are not on immunosuppressive medication.

Most doctors agree that the benefits of the vaccine for people with chronic kidney disease at any stage, those on dialysis, and kidney transplant recipients are much greater than the risk of serious disease or complications from COVID-19. Talk to your doctor or other healthcare professional about getting a COVID-19 vaccine."

Okay, we've heard that before. But what is in the vaccines? According to the Moderna website, there is no virus in the vaccination:

"A vaccine based on messenger RNA (mRNA) technology does not use inactivated virus, attenuated virus, or any other kind of virus.

The Moderna COVID-19 Vaccine uses mRNA to provide a blueprint for your cells to build your body's defense against the virus.

This allows the body to generate an antibody response, and to retain the information in memory immune cells, with the goal of attacking the virus if the vaccinated individual is exposed."

Let's look at Pfizer's vaccine now. This is what the Centers for Disease Control offers:

"All COVID-19 vaccine ingredients are safe. Nearly all of the ingredients in COVID-19 vaccines are ingredients found in many foods – fats, sugars, and salts. The Pfizer-BioNTech COVID-19 vaccine also contains a harmless piece of messenger RNA (mRNA). The COVID-19 mRNA teaches cells in the body how to create an immune response to the virus that causes COVID-19. This response helps protect you from getting sick with COVID-19 in the future.

After the body produces an immune response, it discards all of the vaccine ingredients, just as it would discard any substance that cells no longer need. This process is a part of normal body functioning.

All COVID-19 vaccines are manufactured with as few ingredients as possible and with very small amounts of each ingredient."

I'm not going to research the Johnson & Johnson vaccine since there seems to be some controversy about its effectiveness and the possibility of blood clots. Do not panic if you've taken it, a booster might just do the trick for you. Originally, people liked this vaccine because only one dose was needed.

Vaccines are not your only line of defense. Masks also help. We've been using cloth masks, but the N95 or KN95 seem to provide better protection again the omicron variant.

The FDA explains:

"A surgical mask is a loose-fitting, disposable device that creates a physical barrier between the mouth and nose of the wearer and potential contaminants in the immediate environment. These are often referred to as face masks, although not all face masks are regulated as surgical masks. Note that the edges of the mask are not designed to form a seal around the nose and mouth.

An N95 respirator is a respiratory protective device designed to achieve a very close facial fit and very efficient filtration of airborne particles. Note that the edges of the respirator are designed to form a seal around the nose and mouth. Surgical N95 Respirators are commonly used in healthcare settings and are a subset of N95 Filtering Facepiece Respirators (FFRs), often referred to as N95s."

Let's not forego hand sanitizer, either. We have bottles of it on the shelf right next to our front door. We also have sanitizer in the pockets on the car's doors. We make a conscience effort to use them.

Don't forget about that six foot distance between you and others. Since both my husband and I are immunocompromised, just as you might be if you're a transplantee, we stay home except for medical appointments. And that's only if Televideo appointments are not appropriate. Our visitors are only those who are double vaxxed and boostered. And, yes, we do ask that they wear their masks while in the house and use hand sanitizer upon entering the house.

1/17 *Born with Kidney Disease*

We've had guest blogs from people who donated a kidney, received a preemptive kidney, received a non-preemptive kidney, are on dialysis, and those who advocate for kidney disease awareness. I don't believe we've had a guest blog from someone who was born with kidney disease. That's where Cody Kubiak comes in.

He has his own blog, Kidneys Quit, We Don't. More to the point for us today, Cody was born with kidney disease at a time when kidney transplants were performed on very young children. Well, I'll let him tell his own story:

"Hey there, my name is Cody Kubiak and I have quite the unique kidney transplant story. For starters, unlike many who are diagnosed as they grow older and start having experiences with kidney disease or kidney problems, I was born with kidney failure right from the start. I was born with a rare developmental anomaly known as Posterior Urethral Valves or PUV for short. It's essentially a blockage in your ureters that will kill your kidneys if the blockage isn't fixed. It affects about 1 in every 8,000 male births worldwide. To this day the exact cause isn't known. Nowadays this is fixable in utero but in 1989 that wasn't the case. So, I was born with destroyed kidneys and high blood pressure. I would go on to have ostomies put in and had a couple different bladder surgeries.

My parents even learned how to tube feed me once I eventually left the NICU. To this day I'm still blown away by their ability to handle all they did. The doctors told my parents we'd need to perform a kidney d on me as soon as I was big enough to undergo the procedure. My mother was a match and without any hesitation my mother said let's do it. I had my kidney transplant when I was just 13 months old in April of 1990 thanks to my mom. Nowadays most hospitals won't perform a transplant on anyone that is extremely young like I was. You typically have to wait until you reach a certain weight or age now before transplantation. There's still a lot of debate on the subject on just how young is too young for a transplant.

My childhood was relatively normal. I had good lab numbers mostly and besides the occasional biopsy anytime my creatinine went up I lived what I consider to be a normal life. I thank my parents largely for that because they always found a great balance for me between living a life and being safe. I couldn't play contact sports and had to take meds twice a day everyday but eh, it wasn't bad. I had a great childhood and even into my teen years I went to public school with no problems. I went on to graduate from high school in 2007 and went to community college here in Austin, Texas.

2014 had just started and I had routine labs like always. My creatinine was high which wasn't new to me but meant I needed to undergo a biopsy to see how everything was going. I didn't have any concerns really because my creatinine had fluctuated before and I felt fine. But it was that day I learned that just because you don't feel sick doesn't mean a part of your body isn't. I learned my original kidney trans-plant that I had gotten from my mom was rejecting.

I had heard that term my whole life, but it never clicked with me that it could happen at any time and at any age. Being born into this world put me in a unique position, because I had grown up with this. It's all I knew. I had grown up adapting to it all, but the fear wasn't there because I didn't have the awareness I have because it all happened when I was born. Now after keeping that kidney healthy and safe for years it had enough and I started going through CKD, but this time as a fully aware young adult. I slowly got more and more sick with each month that went by.

By early 2015 my kidney function had fallen low enough to start getting people tested. A good friend of mine started a Facebook group *Cody's Warriors* to help me find a donor. I had several people, friends and family stand up and get tested but they all had some small anomaly that kept them from donating. Fall of 2015 hit and I needed to start dialysis. Just as I was losing hope of finding a donor my aunt, not by blood but through marriage got tested and was a match. On September 16th, 2015, I had my second kidney transplant, and everything went great!

It was after that transplant I wanted to start seeking out others like me and start a blog in hopes of helping others. I felt great and figured everything was behind me, but it wasn't. I started getting sick after the transplant and after months of tests I discovered I had PTLD. [That's Post-transplant lymphoproliferative disease.] Basically, my newly transplanted kidney had the EB virus [Gail here: Epstein-Barr virus infection] my body was never exposed to before. This resulted in Lymphoma cancer. I underwent chemo for about 3 months, and I was in remission. After overcoming all that in 2016, I found out in 2017 I had necrosis in my hip from taking prednisone my whole life. So, I had a complete hip replacement and again overcame and recovered. Then I'd run into the same issue with my left foot and had a bone graft and reconstructive surgery on that in 2019.

Eventually things got better and so far, things have been great. I used to have so much depression over my situation until I started helping people. I found that experience to be infinitely rewarding and my goal today is to just be there for every kidney patient going through even a fraction of this and to see me and understand and know they aren't ever alone no matter what your age is or how you got thrown into this world. If I can do it, so can you."

1/24 *Happy Birthdays*

Next week is my birthday. I'll be three quarters of a century old. Which, of course in my weird way of thinking, brings me to the fact that this month is insulin's 100th birthday. That same insulin that keeps me going now that I have only one third of my pancreas left due to cancer. That same insulin that keeps diabetics, both type 1 and type 2, going. I was curious about how all this came about.

Many thanks to the American Diabetes Association for their comprehensive explanation:

"Before insulin was discovered in 1921, people with diabetes didn't live for long; there wasn't much doctors could do for them. The most effective treatment was to put patients with diabetes on very strict diets with minimal carbohydrate intake. This could buy patients a few extra years but couldn't save them. Harsh diets (some prescribed as little as 450 calories a day!) sometimes even caused patients to die of starvation.

So how did this wonderful breakthrough blossom? Let's travel back a little more than 100 years ago....

In 1889, two German researchers, Oskar Minkowski and Joseph von Mering, found that when the pancreas gland was removed from dogs, the animals developed symptoms of diabetes and died soon afterward. This led to the idea that the pancreas was the site where 'pancreatic substances' (insulin) were produced. Later experimenters narrowed this search to the islets of Langerhans (a fancy name for clusters of specialized cells in the pancreas). In 1910, Sir Edward Albert Sharpey-Shafer suggested only one chemical was missing from the pancreas in people with diabetes. He decided to call this chemical insulin, which comes for the Latin word insula, meaning "island."

So, what happened next? Something truly miraculous. In 1921, a young surgeon named Frederick Banting and his assistant Charles Best figured out how to remove insulin from a dog's pancreas. Skeptical colleagues said the stuff looked like 'thick brown muck,' but little did they know this would lead to life and hope for millions of people with diabetes.

With this murky concoction, Banting and Best kept another dog with severe diabetes alive for 70 days—the dog died only when there was no more extract. With this success, the researchers, along with the help of colleagues J.B. Collip and John Macleod, went a step further. A more refined and pure form of insulin was developed, this time from the pancreases of cattle.

In January 1922, Leonard Thompson, a 14-year-old boy dying from diabetes in a Toronto hospital, became the first person to receive an injection of insulin. Within 24 hours, Leonard's dangerously high blood glucose levels dropped to near-normal levels.

The news about insulin spread around the world like wildfire. In 1923, Banting and Macleod received the Nobel Prize in Medicine, which they shared with Best and Collip. Thank you, diabetes researchers!

Soon after, the medical firm Eli Lilly started large-scale production of insulin. It wasn't long before there was enough insulin to supply the entire North American continent. In the decades to follow, manufacturers developed a variety of slower-acting insulins, the first introduced by Novo Nordisk Pharmaceuticals, Inc., in 1936.

Insulin from cattle and pigs was used for many years to treat diabetes and saved millions of lives, but it wasn't perfect, as it caused allergic reactions in many patients. The first genetically engineered, synthetic 'human' insulin was produced in 1978 using E. coli bacteria to produce the insulin. Eli Lilly went on in 1982 to sell the first commercially available biosynthetic human insulin under the brand name Humulin.

Insulin now comes in many forms, from regular human insulin identical to what the body produces on its own, to ultra-rapid and ultra-long acting insulins. Thanks to decades of research, people with diabetes can choose from a variety of formulas and ways to take their insulin based on their personal needs and lifestyles. From Humalog to Novolog and insulin pens to pumps, insulin has come a long way. It may not be a cure for diabetes, but it's literally a life saver."

Naturally, I had to know who I recognized that might have died from diabetes or diabetes related complications. Ranker.com was helpful here:

Alexander Graham Bell in 1922

Johnny Cash in 2003

Carroll O'Connor in 2011

Buddy Hackett in 2003 [Personal note, I remember seeing him perform while I was a cocktail waitress in one of the Catskill Mountain Borsch Belt hotels where I earned my college tuition.]

James Cagney in 1986

Ella Fitzgerald in 1996

Penny Marshall in 2018

Jules Verne in 1905

Nell Carter in 2003

William F. Buckley, Jr. in 2008

Okay, I get it that Mr. Bell and Mr. Verne died before insulin was in common use, but what did the others die of? According to the *New York Times*, Mr. Cagney not only had diabetes, but had suffered several strokes. The *Los Angeles Times* tells us that Ms. Fitzgerald died of heart disease and stroke. I went to the *Tennessean* to discover that Mr. Cash died of respiratory failure brought on by complications from diabetes. The *Washington Post* mentions that Mr. Hackett had diabetes. The *New York Post* points out that Ms. Carter had suffered from diabetes for years. The *Guardian* explained that Mr. Buckley suffered from diabetes and emphysema. Wikipedia informs us that Mr. O'Connor died of a heart attack brought on by complications from diabetes. Ms. Marshall died of atherosclerotic cardiovascular disease and diabetes according to *USA Today*.

My point? Diabetes doesn't exist in a vacuum. If not taken care of, there can be other comorbidities that seem to sneak in. We know that high blood glucose can damage your small blood vessels, including those in the kidneys. It's the kidneys that filter your blood. If your kidneys are not working properly - perhaps due to diabetes damage – fluids and wastes build up in your body. A body that doesn't function as well as it could will lead to other illnesses.

Take care of your diabetes. Work with your endocrinologist to find the correct dosage and brand of insulin you need... and be thankful for insulin. I know I certainly am.

1/31 *Skin Deep*

Holy Cow! It's the last day of January already. One down, 11 more to go. That's quite a bit of time to get 2022 to be different from 2020 [As Natalie Gelman sings] and 2021. Do we ever need that to happen.

For example, I had a dermatology appointment recently. Before I exited my car, I made sure my N95 was in place and hang what my hair looked up with those straps mangling it. Then, I approached the no contact thermometer. No fever. Great, now I could stand six feet away from the person in front of me waiting to check in. Once she was done, I was handed a freshly cleaned iPad upon which to check in. The waiting room was enormous… and there were exactly three people waiting. Finally, it was my turn.

I had just enough time to start wondering what, if anything, chronic kidney disease had to do with the condition of your skin. Well, that was one good thing; due to the pandemic, there's now a very short waiting time to see your doctor. [I'd rather go back to long waits and no pandemic.]

One thing I remembered about CKD and your skin was that once you have a transplant, you are more vulnerable to skin cancer. In fact, a transplanted friend just when through this. Apparently, his sun hat and sun block weren't enough. Now he uses zinc oxide on his nose, too. Come to think of it, he's the second person I know personally who's gone through this.

What else? Are there other connections between CKD and your skin? Let's find out.

New-Medical, Life Sciences, which is based in the UK and Australia, taught me a new word and, unfortunately, a new condition:

"Xerosis

Xerosis is a condition that is characterized by dry and rough skin. The patient usually experiences scaling, fissures, and general discomfort. About 50-75% of dialysis patients experience this particular skin issue. The cracks that can develop in the skin increases the chance for further infection from viruses or bacteria present in the environment.

Management of xerosis includes:

Emollients: Moisturizers and emollients can soothe dry, scaly skin.

Avoiding hot water and humidifiers: Too much hot water can further aggravate skin issues and cause excess drying.

Bath oils: Bathing in natural oils can further moisturize the skin.

Steroid cream: Medical creams can help alleviate itching."

I have seen this, but living in Arizona, presumed it was from too much exposure to the sun. As you can see, I learn as much as you do by writing these blogs.

I decided to turn to some of my usual search sites. **Medscape** did not disappoint, although we will need a vocabulary lesson with this information.:

"Pigmentary alteration occurs in 25-70% of the dialysis population and increases over time. A multitude of uremia-related changes are responsible for the pigmentary alterations. Before the widespread use of erythropoietin, pallor was common and was attributed to the significant anemia. A brown–to–slate-gray discoloration may occur as a result of **hemosiderin** deposition in association with iron overload from excessive transfusions. Over time, many patients develop a yellowish hue, which has been attributed to retained **urochromes** and **carotene**, which are subsequently deposited in the epidermis and subcutaneous tissues. A brownish hyperpigmentation is common, mostly in a sun-exposed distribution. This hyperpigmentation results from an increase in melanin production because of an increase in poorly dialyzable **beta-melanocyte stimulating hormone.**"

Now for that vocabulary lesson. I bolded the words above that will be defined below.

Hemosiderin: "Hemosiderin staining is a medical condition in which one presents yellow or brown patches on the skin. These are in fact the result of the macrophages [Gail here: these are a type of white blood cell] consuming the dead red blood cells, leading to the production of hemosiderin." [MDDK.com]

Urochrome: "a yellow pigment to which the color of normal urine is principally due." [Merriam-Webster Dictionary]

Carotene: "Yellow-red pigments widely distributed in plants and animals, notably in carrots; include precursors of vitamin A." [Medical Dictionary for the Dental Professions]

Beta-melanocyte stimulating hormone: "The major biological property of b-Melanocyte Stimulating Hormone is hyperpigmentation." [InterScience Institute]

There's another way that CKD affects your skin. Have you heard the term pruritus? We know the suffix 'us' means prone to, but what about 'prur'? ETYMOLOGEEK tells us,

"English word pruritus comes from Proto-Indo-European *prews-, and later Latin prurio (I itch or tingle. I long for.)" Apologies for that sidestep. Old English teachers never die, you know. Let's get back on track.

DermNet Az tells us that pruritus means,

"Pruritus is the medical term for itch. Itch is an unpleasant sensation on the skin that provokes the desire to rub or scratch the area to obtain relief. Itch can cause discomfort and frustration; in severe cases it can lead to disturbed sleep, anxiety and depression. Constant scratching to obtain relief can damage the skin (excoriation, lichenification) and reduce its effectiveness as a major protective barrier.

Pruritus is often a symptom of an underlying disease process such as a skin problem, a systemic disease, or abnormal nerve impulses."

CKD is a systemic disease.

How about one more? Moon face is a term often used instead of the medical term moon facies. MedicineNet elucidates,

"Moon face, otherwise known as moon facies, is a medical sign characterized by the face developing a rounded appearance due to fat deposits on the sides of the face.

The most common cause of moon face is said to be associated with Cushing's syndrome or prolonged steroid treatment (especially corticosteroids). "

Healthline further explains,

"One of the most common causes of moon face is the steroid medication prednisone. Prednisone is prescribed for a variety of conditions because it helps reduce swelling and inflammation.

You might be prescribed prednisone if you've had an organ transplant...."

That includes kidney transplants.

You know that old song,

"Your thigh bone connected to your hip bone
Your hip bone connected to your backbone"?

Well, it turns out your inner organs are connected to your outer organ, too. Hey, did you know that your skin is the largest organ?

2/7 **The Hard Stuff**

With marijuana being legalized in so many states and so much information about it more readily available, I started wondering what other drugs might do to chronic kidney disease patients. I don't mean prescriptions, but substances like heroin or cocaine. So, I did what I always do: I researched it. I have a curious mind.

The National Kidney Foundation tells us in no uncertain terms,

"Most street drugs, including heroin, cocaine and ecstasy can cause high blood pressure, stroke, heart failure and even death, in some cases from only one use. Cocaine, heroin and amphetamines also can cause kidney damage."

I wanted to know how they can do this and learned a new word in the process. This is from The Recovery Village, a rehabilitation center:

"Essentially what happens with rhabdomyolysis is a breakdown of tissue during an overdose-related coma because the person has been not moving for an extended period. The muscles start to disintegrate and that produces chemicals, which then go into the bloodstream and set off other damaging reactions throughout the organs. This is one of the number one reasons for kidney failure. During this situation, heart damage and heart attack can also occur.

Also, people who use heroin intravenously may be more likely to contract infections that can lead to kidney inflammation, and for people who inject heroin under the skin, there's an increased chance of getting secondary amyloidosis. This is a buildup of protein in organs and tissues that can lead to kidney failure."

By the way, you're right if you guess the new word is rhabdomyolysis. Amyloid may be another word you need defined since it's helpful in understanding the definition of amyloidosis. That's what the Merriam-Webster Dictionary is for:

"a waxy translucent substance consisting primarily of protein that is deposited in some animal organs and tissues under abnormal conditions (such as Alzheimer's disease)"

Worser and worser, as I image Alice from **Alice in Wonderland** might say. But we're not done yet, DrugAbuse.com explains why street drugs are even worse for us as CKD patients than we may have thought:

"Drugs and alcohol are no exception when it comes to the renal filtration process; in fact, the majority of abused substances are excreted through the kidneys ....

There are a few factors that influence the kidneys' ability to expel drugs, such as...:

The acidity of urine.

The kidneys' condition.

Circulation through kidneys.

Urine flow.

Kidney functioning can be negatively impacted by....:

Exposure to toxins.

Aging.

Hypertension.

Diabetes.

Persistent kidney infections.

Nephrolithiasis (kidney stones).

In some cases, if the kidneys are not functioning properly, the effects of a drug may be amplified and thus, the kidneys are more easily prone to toxicity from the substance.... This can be particularly dangerous for someone suffering from an addiction to drugs or alcohol who is often increasing their dose to counteract tolerance."

So, it's not just using street drugs that's dangerous for our kidneys. It's also that the more you use street drugs, the more you need for the high you seek. That further damages your kidneys.

In some instances, these street drugs can cause kidney disease in people who had normal kidneys before the use of street drugs. This is from the American Addiction Centers,

"Drug abuse can also impact the functioning of the kidneys. If the kidneys are not functioning properly, the effects of drug use can be amplified, and this can lead to further issues with the kidneys. For instance, individuals who develop tolerance to alcohol or drugs often significantly increase the amount of the substances they use, and this can contribute to problems with toxicity and kidney functioning over time.

Chronic abuse of drugs or alcohol can lead to severe kidney damage and even to kidney failure. Substance abuse may directly damage the kidneys or may indirectly damage them through some other process, such as increased body temperature or rhabdomyolysis (the breakdown of muscle tissue in the release of cells in the bloodstream)."

Hmmm, that could mean that if you didn't have CKD when you started using street drugs, you may develop it by using these street drugs. To make it worse, it's not always CKD, which is a decline in your kidney function for at least three months. Street drugs can also cause Acute Kidney Injury [AKI], which is defined by MedScape as:

"..., is commonly defined as an abrupt decline in renal function, clinically manifesting as a reversible acute increase in nitrogen waste products—measured by blood urea nitrogen (BUN) and serum creatinine levels—over the course of hours to weeks."

Hours to weeks. It doesn't take long for street drugs to affect your kidneys in some cases.

Another treatment center, Sunrise House Treatment Center has some interesting information about street drugs and what they do to our kidneys,

"Some drugs of abuse can damage the kidneys more than others. Here are some substances that cause kidney damage or renal failure:

.... Benzodiazepines: When abused, these psychiatric prescription medications can cause rhabdomyolysis, or the breakdown of muscles that damages the kidneys.

Cocaine: This potent stimulant can lead to rhabdomyolysis, or the breakdown of muscle tissue that poisons the blood and eventually the kidneys. The drug is toxic to the kidneys in multiple other ways, usually involving blood circulation through the organs and how the kidneys are able to filter out toxins to convert to urine. People who abuse cocaine for a long time are much more likely to suffer kidney damage or renal failure than the general public.

.... MDMA: This club drug can cause kidney failure from dehydration, chemical adulterants, and hyperthermia (overheating), leading to muscle breakdown.

Methamphetamines: Crystal meth and other versions of methamphetamines break down muscles and release toxins into the system that the kidneys cannot filter properly.

Opioids: Heroin is especially toxic to the kidneys, in part due to the adulterants found in this street drug. However, any opioid drug can cause damage to the kidneys through muscle breakdown.

Synthetic marijuana: Kidney damage can occur rapidly due to toxins in any synthetic drug, but it can occur particularly quickly due to abuse of synthetic cannabinoids like K2 or Spice. These lab-created chemicals are similar in structure to cannabinoids like THC, but they do not have the same effects on the brain. Because they are made with artificial chemicals, there are many other molecules in them that can be very harmful to the body. Additionally, these unregulated drugs contain vastly different doses of the intoxicating substance, so dosing is nearly impossible, which can rapidly lead to overdose. Kidney failure is one consequence of overdosing on synthetic marijuana."

Notice it's *synthetic* marijuana that can cause kidney damage. But I think I'll continue to get my high from watching my grandson's antics anyway.

2/14 *The Big House (and the Little House)*

My readers tell me the most interesting things. A comment on last week's blog about street drugs led me to research chronic kidney disease in the incarcerated population. I presumed it was going to be a difficult search for material since it seemed somewhat esoteric to me. Was I ever wrong. My first inquiry brought up the following.

Oh wait, first we need to make certain you know that jail and prison are two separate things. Let's turn to the Merriam-Webster Dictionary. You didn't expect any other, did you?

"If you wish to avoid ambiguity in use you should use prison for serious crimes with longer sentences, and jail for less serious crimes, or for detention awaiting trial. And penitentiary, when referring to a hoosegow, often has the specific meaning of 'a state or federal prison in the U.S.'"

Incarceration usually refers to long term detention, in other words, prison.

Okay, now we can turn the prison population. An article in The Clinical Journal of the American Society of Nephrology stated in no uncertain terms,

"CKD affects 15% of US adults and is associated with higher morbidity and mortality. CKD disproportionately affects certain populations, including racial and ethnic minorities and individuals from disadvantaged socioeconomic backgrounds. These groups are also disproportionately affected by incarceration and barriers to accessing health services. Incarceration represents an opportunity to link marginalized individuals to CKD care. Despite a legal obligation to provide a community standard of care including the screening and treatment of individuals with CKD, there is little evidence to suggest systematic efforts are in place to address this prevalent, costly, and ultimately fatal condition."

Did that mean the prisoners with CKD weren't treated? Or that they weren't screened? And if so, why not? It couldn't be that CKD was ignored and allowed to progress until prisoners died, could it? I was becoming more and more curious about this. Back to the internet.

Medicare usually pays for dialysis. Here's what Medicare has to say about medical coverage while you're incarcerated.

"If you had Medicare before your arrest, you will remain eligible for the program while you are incarcerated. However, Medicare generally will not pay for your medical care. Instead your correctional facility will provide and pay for your care. Once you are released, Medicare will resume coverage if you remained enrolled."

According to the Federal Bureau of Prisons,

"The Bureau's professional staff provides essential medical, dental, and mental health (psychiatric) services in a manner consistent with accepted community standards for a correctional environment. The Bureau uses licensed and credentialed health care providers in its ambulatory care units, which are supported by community consultants and specialists. For inmates with chronic or acute medical conditions, the Bureau operates several medical referral centers providing advanced care.

CKD is a systemic disease.

How about one more? Moon face is a term often used instead of the medical term moon facies. MedicineNet elucidates,

"Moon face, otherwise known as moon facies, is a medical sign characterized by the face developing a rounded appearance due to fat deposits on the sides of the face.

Health promotion is emphasized through counseling provided during examinations, education about the effects of medications, infectious disease prevention and education, and chronic care clinics for conditions such as cardiovascular disease, diabetes, and hypertension. The Bureau promotes environ-mental health for staff and inmates alike through its emphasis on a clean-air environment and the maintenance of safe conditions in inmate living and work areas. The Bureau's food service program emphasizes heart-healthy diets, nutrition education, and dietary counseling in conjunction with certain medical treatment."

While I found the protocols for dealing with hypertension and diabetes on this website - the two leading causes of CKD - I didn't find any for dealing with kidney disease itself.

So, I looked further and found myself reading an October 2020 article in Transplantation.

"The US Constitution guarantees adequate medical care to all convicts… however, transplantation is considered ethically contentious…. The determination to authorize transplantation for an inmate is often made by the prison administration on a case-by-case basis. Nevertheless, the Organ Procurement and Transplantation Network's ethics committee advises that 'one's status as a prisoner should not preclude them from consideration for a transplant….' However, Organ Procurement and Transplantation Network acknowledges that other nonmedical factors may influence patient's candidacy for transplant and delegates the listing decisions to the individual transplant programs…. Consequently, programs make listing decisions in the absence of uniform criteria and hesitate to evaluate and waitlist prisoners…. The possible reasons are logistic challenges in clinical care, security concerns, uncertainty regarding adherence and concern of loss of follow-up.

Overcoming these challenges requires program's personnel to be highly motivated to accept convicts for transplantation."

Well, what about jails? How do they deal with chronic conditions? I discovered a site called Health Affairs that explained,

"In 2019, there were a total of 10.3 million jail admissions with an average daily census of 741,900 across the United States. With a mean stay of 26 days, care for chronic medical conditions can be interrupted, jeopardizing the health and well-being of the incarcerated individual. Additionally, one in four jailed individuals will be arrested again, and these periodic short stays in jail introduce chaos into ongoing medical care. This is particularly concerning because the incarcerated population has a higher prevalence of chronic conditions such as diabetes mellitus, hypertension, and asthma compared to the general population...."

2/21 *Black History Month and the Present*

I'll bet you thought I'd forgotten all about Black History Month. Not at all, dear readers, not at all. It's just that since this is a yearly occurrence and I've been blogging about kidney disease for 14 years, it becomes harder and harder to uncover Black nephrologists I haven't written about before. Of course, including current Black nephrologists changes the picture somewhat. This year, I turned to Blackamericanweb for some help and found it,

"Dr. Velma Scantlebury [Gail here: sometimes she is referred to as Scantlebury-White.] is the first African American female transplant surgeon in America. She is currently the associate director of the Kidney Transplant Program at Christiana Care in Delaware. [Gail here again: actually, she retired last year.] With more than 200 live donor kidney transplants under her career, she holds extensive research credit in African American kidney donation led by Northwestern Medicine Transplantation Surgeon Dinee C. Simpson, MD, Dr. Scantlebury has stated that she refuses to retire until there are ten more Black women in transplant surgery in the United States. Currently there is only one other Black woman transplant surgeon."

And who is the other 'Black woman transplant surgeon'? Could it be the Dinee C. Simpson mentioned above? I went to Northwestern Medicine's site to find out.

"The Northwestern Medicine African American Transplant Access Program (AATAP) … is committed to breaking down barriers to transplant care in the African American community through access to education, resources and world-class transplant care. Dr. Simpson, who is the first African American female transplant surgeon in Illinois, founded the program to address disparity in access to transplantation experienced by the Black community."

Nice, but two Black nephrologists do not a blog make. Thankfully, Black Health Matters came to the rescue:

"Kirk Campbell, M.D.

An associate professor in the Division of Nephrology and the Vice Chair of Diversity and Inclusion, as well as the director of the Nephrology Fellowship Program and an ombudsperson for medical students at the Icahn School of Medicine at Mount Sinai in New York. Kirk Campbell, M.D., treats patients with renal disease and leads an NIH-funded research program focused on understanding the mechanism of podocyte injury in the progression of proteinuric kidney diseases....

Olayiwola Ayodeji, M.D.

Nephrologist Olayiwola Ayodeji, M.D., has led the development of the Clinical Trials Program at Peninsula Kidney Associates and served as a principal investigator on many research trials. He currently serves as the Medical Director of Davita Newmarket Dialysis Center and the Davita Home Training Center. He is board certified in nephrology and internal medicine.

Paul W. Crawford, M.D.

A nephrology and hypertension specialist with a private practice in Chicago, Paul W. Crawford, M.D. has been practicing for more than 40 years. He is a graduate of Loyola University of Chicago/Stritch School of Medicine.

Crystal Gadegbeku, M.D.

A graduate of the University of Virginia, Crystal Gadegbeku, M.D., is a nephrology specialist in Philadelphia, Pennsylvania. She is Chief of the section of nephrology, hypertension and kidney transplantation, and Vice Chair of community outreach at Lewis Katz School of Medicine at Temple University. Her clinical interests include chronic kidney disease, hypertension in chronic kidney disease and pregnancy in chronic kidney disease.

Eddie Greene, M.D.

Mayo Clinic internist and nephrologist Eddie Green, M.D., treats chronic kidney disease, heart disease and kidney cancer. His interests include chronic renal failure, cardiovascular disease in chronic renal failure and renal cell cancer.

Susanne Nicholas, M.D.

Board certified in internal medicine and nephrology, Susanne Nicholas, M.D., has clinical interests in nephrology and hypertension. Her research over the past 15-plus years has led to the identification of a novel biomarker of diabetic kidney disease, which is being validated in clinical studies.

Carmen Peralta, M.D.

Clinical investigator and association professor of medicine Carmen Peralta, M.D., is co-founder and executive director of the Kidney Health Research Collaborative. She is a leader in the epidemiology of kidney disease and hypertension. A graduate of Johns Hopkins University, her research activity focuses on three areas: 1) approaches to improving care of people with kidney disease and reducing racial and ethnic disparities; 2) hypertension, arterial stiffness and kidney disease; and 3) biomarkers for detection, classification and risk of early kidney disease.

Neil Powe, M.D.

A graduate of Harvard Medical School, Neal Powe, M.D., is head of the University of California San Francisco Medicine Service at the Priscilla Chan and Mark Zuckerberg San Francisco General Hospital. This is one of the leading medicine departments in a public hospital with strong basic, clinical and health services research programs focused on major diseases affecting diverse patients locally, nationally and globally. His primary intellectual pursuits involve kidney disease patient-oriented research, epidemiology and outcomes and effectiveness research.

Crystal Tyson, M.D.

Located in Durham, North Carolina, Crystal Tyson, M.D., is a specialist in nephrology and renal medicine. "I enjoy building relationships with my patients and collaborating with them on how to best accomplish those goals with available therapies," she says.

As you can see, the Black community is currently represented in the field of nephrology. It might have been that the history of Black nephrologists was limited by not only race, but how new the field was. We need to remember that nephrology was not recognized as a specialty until the 1950s.

However, Zippa.com: the Career Expert, had what I consider distressing news on their site. Last year, only 4.6% of nephrologists were Black, down from 5.21% in 2016. Could that be because Blacks were the lowest paid nephrologists? And why are they still the lowest paid nephrologists? I find this disturbing. Don't you?

2/28 *My Friend's Wife*

I live in Arizona. Therefore, it's almost a default that I know undocumented immigrants. I met many DREAMers when I was teaching at Phoenix College. The American Immigration Council tells us:

"The first version of the Development, Relief, and Education for Alien Minors (DREAM) Act was introduced in 2001. In part because of the publicity around that bill, young undocumented immigrants have been referred to as 'Dreamers.' Over the last 20 years, at least 11 versions of the Dream Act have been introduced in Congress. While the various versions of the bill have contained some key differences, they all would have provided a pathway to legal status for undocumented people who came to this country as children. Some versions have garnered as many as 48 co-sponsors in the U.S. Senate and 152 in the House of Representatives.

Despite bipartisan support for each iteration of the bill, none have become law. To date, the 2010 bill came closest to full passage when it passed the House but fell just five votes short of the 60 needed to proceed in the Senate."

And then, there's DACA or Deferred Action for Childhood Arrivals. According to U.S. Citizenship and Immigration Services:

"On June 15, 2012, the secretary of Homeland Security announced that certain people who came to the United States as children and meet several guidelines may request consideration of deferred action for a period of two years, subject to renewal. They are also eligible for work authorization. Deferred action is a use of prosecutorial discretion to defer removal action against an individual for a certain period of time. Deferred action does not provide lawful status."

Not only did I meet students who were undocumented immigrants, but also everyday workers in my life. Now here's where we get to kidney disease and undocumented immigrants. One such person that I've known for many years knew that I'm a chronic kidney disease awareness advocate. I know very little Spanish, and his English is somewhat limited. In our stilted way, we discussed that his wife is on dialysis. I wondered how this was possible since they are both undocumented.

It turns out that Arizona is one of only twelve states that offer non-emergency dialysis to undocumented immigrants. OMG. Does that mean that all the other states allow them to die if they need dialysis? Well, not exactly. The National Center for Biotechnology Information explains:

"Standard of care for people with kidney failure is thrice-weekly outpatient hemodialysis, daily peritoneal or home hemodialysis, or kidney transplantation. Undocumented immigrants are excluded from the provisions of the Affordable Care Act, the diagnosis-based 1972 Medicare End-Stage Renal Disease entitlement program, and a range of federally funded Medicaid programs that pay for standard outpatient dialysis. The Emergency Medical Treatment and Active Labor Act requires hospitals to treat anyone who enters with an emergency medical condition, enabling undocumented immigrants to receive dialysis when they present to hospitals with emergency indications....

Emergency-only dialysis is associated with lower quality of life, high symptom burden, and significant anxiety about death.... Compared with people receiving standard dialysis, this population's 5-year mortality is 14-fold higher and they spend more time in the hospital and less time in the outpatient setting.... Emergency-only dialysis is taxing on the health care system. Studies show that their providers experience emotional exhaustion and burnout from the perception of propagating unjust, unethical, and substandard medical care.... It is also extremely costly: emergency-only dialysis costs $285,000 to $400,000 per person per year... compared with $76,177 to $90,971 per person per year for standard dialysis.... Switching from emergency-only dialysis to outpatient dialysis is associated with a cost reduction of $5,768 per person per month...."

This is sounding dismal. I asked my friend about a transplant for his wife. He explained that wasn't possible. They couldn't afford it. I wasn't sure what he meant so I decided to find out since he couldn't explain more than that. Weren't there governmental agencies that would help financially? The news is not good. This is what KidneyNews offers:

"The policy of the Organ Procurement and Transplantation Network (OPTN) clearly states that 'deceased donor organ allocation to candidates for transplantation shall not differ on the basis of the candidate's residency or citizenship status in the United States.'

There appears to be no legislation barring undocumented immigrants from receiving organs, but the lack of federally funded health insurance achieves that end, resulting in automatic and indirect exclusion. The Omnibus Budget Reconciliation Act passed by Congress in 1986 prohibits the use of federal Medicaid funding for payment of care provided to undocumented immigrants except for what qualifies as emergency medical care under the Emergency Medical Treatment and Active Labor Act (EMTALA).

In 1996, further legislation denied all state and local public benefits to undocumented immigrants and left the states to pass their own laws to determine the eligibility criteria under which public benefits would be available to undocumented immigrants. Additional legislation was passed to augment federal Medicaid funding to states with the greatest number of undocumented immigrants. Undocumented immigrants with catastrophic illnesses such as kidney failure, cancer, or traumatic brain injuries are also excluded from the Patient Protection and Affordable Care Act.

Under EMTALA, all states must offer at least emergent-only dialysis to all patients; however, kidney transplantation is not considered to be part of this program and is not offered to undocumented immigrants...."

Of course, there are all kinds of ethical issues here, but today I'm just writing about my friend's wife's life... and I am heartbroken that this wife, mother, and grandmother will not be able to procure a kidney because she is undocumented. Yes, this may be an insurance issue, but it still means no kidney for this woman.

3/7 Say It Out Loud

I have a cousin I'm very friendly with who loves being a member of Toastmasters International. She's been involved with them for years and years. Her opinion of them is that they help you express your message and that it's fun. That, of course, got me to thinking. I wondered if Toastmasters could be useful in advocating for a transplant, especially your own transplant.

Talk about serendipity! It was just about at this point in time that Leesa Thompson and I got to communicating. She'd had a transplant fairly recently and had been thinking along the same lines I was. One thing led to another, and I asked her if she would guest blog about her experience. She, in turn, approached Josiah Wolfson who explains why he joined the Virtual Kidney Stories Toastmasters Club. I find this exciting. What if all those that wanted transplants could advocate for themselves effectively? Let's see what Josiah and Leesa, who worked together on this blog, have to say.

(Josiah is the Vice-President in charge of Public Relations for the club. Leesa is the President.)

JOIN THE VIRTUAL KIDNEY STORIES TOASTMASTERS CLUB AND IMPROVE YOUR ADVOCACY

"Your ability to advocate for yourself may determine whether you live or die."

As a patient living with kidney disease, it may feel like you're on your own. From one day to the next, you go from living your normal life to being diagnosed with an unfamiliar disease that rocks your world. It's normal for things to get harder before they get easier and that can be overwhelming. Unfortunately, you can't expect the system to work for you. You're better off hoping for the best while expecting the worst. Taking the initiative by (a) getting clear on your treatment options and (b) advocating for yourself is the best way to improve your circumstances.

There's no guarantee that anyone will provide you with a comprehensive overview of your treatment options. So, you have to educate yourself. Spoiler alert, dialysis and kidney transplantation are the only two treatment options for kidney disease. It is undisputed that kidney transplantation is the better option for those patients healthy enough for the operation, but that requires a kidney donation.

Advocating for yourself will take different forms at different times. It spans from fighting to be added to the UNOS Kidney Transplant Waitlist, to asking someone to consider becoming your lifesaving kidney donor. Putting yourself out there like this may scare you and will likely push you outside your comfort zone. These fears and insecurities stop more than half of kidney patients from asking someone to be a living kidney donor. Your ability to advocate for yourself may determine whether you live or die.

Leesa Thompson, a recent kidney recipient, partnered with Toastmasters to create the Kidney Stories Toastmasters Club, a dedicated Toastmasters club focused on the kidney community. Leesa had experienced the empowering benefits of Toastmasters in a general community club that helped her find her voice to advocate for herself.

Leesa went from battling chronic kidney disease for more than four decades to getting a lifesaving kidney transplant. By developing her advocate skills, she found a non-directed kidney donor within eight months of being informed that she would need to begin dialysis if she didn't get a kidney transplant. Through social media, yard signs, newspaper articles, a magazine spread, an alumni spotlight, flyers, and calling cards, Leesa's online story received over 32,500 views in only six weeks. Her efforts resulted in a stranger becoming her swap donor. Leesa has been a member of Toastmasters for sixteen months. She credits her improved public speaking, leadership skills, and heightened motivation to help others to Toastmasters.

Leesa asked me to join the Kidney Stories Toastmasters Club and shared with me her vision of using the time-tested Toastmasters program to help the kidney community. The club mission is to provide a supportive and positive learning experience in which members of the kidney community are empowered to develop communication and leadership skills, resulting in greater self-confidence and personal growth in order to better advocate for themselves and others.

Toastmasters International is a longstanding nonprofit organization that helps people find their voice in a safe space. Through its educational program and regular small group peer driven meetings, Toastmasters brings benefits such as:

- Improved communication, public speaking, leadership, and soft skills;
- Sharpened presentational skills;
- More confident members who can think better on their feet; and
- Increased team collaboration and networking.

I'm Josiah Wolfson and I joined the Kidney Stories Club because I want to help create a safe space for those in the kidney community to share their stories while also improving my own leadership and advocacy skills. On January 13, 2022, I donated a kidney to a stranger. I saw it as a simple cost benefit analysis that provided low risk of surgical or long-term complications and a couple weeks of recovery in exchange for saving a life. Sharing my transplant story publicly proved more challenging than the transplant itself. I created Kidney Abundance @kidneyabundance) to promote living kidney donation because we could collectively solve the kidney shortage crisis if more people would donate a kidney. I feel fortunate to have the opportunity use my voice to advocate for such an important cause. Since joining the Kidney Stories Club, I have already had the opportunity to share my transplant story, receive constructive feedback about my speech, and network with others from the kidney community. The support and accountability I have received from the Kidney Stories Toastmasters Club has encouraged me to continue spreading my story.

Join the Kidney Stories Toastmasters Club and see that you are not alone in your battle against kidney disease. Our virtual meetings are at 7:00-8:30pm (EST) and will be held every first and third Sunday of the month. Take this important step in developing skills to craft and deliver a persuasive speech that may just save your life. Email kidneystoriestoastmasters@gmail.com for the zoom link and membership information.

Gail here. Consider this... and then send your email. If I needed a transplant, I certainly would.

3/14 *It's the Month of....*

World Kidney Day was March 10th this year. While I publicized it widely on social media, I didn't blog about it because I have just about every year for the last 11 years or so. Just scroll to 'World Kidney Day' on the topics dropdown to the right of the blog and you can read last year's blog about it.

By now, we all know March is National Kidney Month as well as Women's History Month. Did you know it's also National Nutrition Month? National Day Calendar tells us there is much more being celebrated this month:

"Asset Management Awareness Month

Developmental Disabilities Awareness Month

Endometriosis Awareness Month

Irish-American Heritage Month

Multiple Sclerosis Awareness Month

National Athletic Training Month

National Brain Injury Awareness Month

National Breast Implant Awareness Month

National Caffeine Awareness Month

National Celery Month

National Cerebral Palsy Awareness Month

National Cheerleading Safety Month

National Craft Month

National Colorectal Cancer Awareness Month

National Credit Education Month

National Flour Month

National Frozen Food Month

National Kidney Month

National Noodle Month

National Nutrition Month

National Peanut Month

National Sauce Month

National Trisomy Awareness Month

National Umbrella Month

National Women's History Month

National Social Work Month"

I'll admit I had to look up Trisomy. I figured it was three something since tri means three. The Medical Dictionary backed me up:

"the presence of an additional (third) chromosome of one type in an otherwise diploid cell (2n +1)."

Now, I'll agree with you that some of these seem pretty silly, but I also think it's no accident that National Kidney Month and National Nutrition Month are both in March. I haven't written about the basics of chronic kidney disease treatment in a while, but nutrition is one of them. I'll let the National Kidney Foundation explain about the first of the '3 Ps and 1 S' as I called them in my first CKD book, **What Is It and How Did I Get It? Early Stage Chronic Kidney Disease**.

"Protein

Your body needs protein to help build muscle, repair tissue, and fight infection. If you have kidney disease, you may need to watch how much protein you eat. Having too much protein can cause waste to build up in your blood, and your kidneys may not be able to remove all the extra waste. If protein intake is too low, however, it may cause other problems so it is essential to eat the right amount each day.

The amount of protein you need is based on:

your body size

your kidney problem

the amount of protein in your urine

Your dietitian or healthcare provider can tell you how much protein you should eat."

My first nephrologist limited me to 5 ounces of protein daily 13 years ago. That still hasn't changed.

What about that one S? I thought the National Kidney Fund would be helpful here and they were, as long as you remember sodium, the 1 S, is one of the two elements of table salt:

"Salt makes you thirsty and can make your body retain fluid. Having more fluid in your body can raise your blood pressure. When you have high blood pressure, your kidneys must work harder to filter blood. Over time, this can lead to kidney damage.

Too much fluid in your body also puts more strain on your heart, lowers your protein levels, and leads to difficulty breathing. Taking steps to limit excess fluid buildup, and thereby controlling blood pressure, is vital to improving your health.

If you have high blood pressure, eating a low or no added salt diet can help to lower it. Increasing your daily physical activity and taking blood pressure medicines if prescribed by your doctor are other ways to manage your blood pressure. Taking steps to keep your blood pressure at a healthy level may help keep kidney disease from getting worse."2 Ps to go. One of them is potassium. I went right to my old and trusted site WebMD for information:

"Every time you eat a banana or a baked potato with the skin on (not just the tasty buttered insides), you're getting potassium. This essential mineral keeps your muscles healthy and your heartbeat and blood pressure steady.

If you have a heart or kidney condition, though, your doctor may recommend a low-potassium diet. Your kidneys are responsible for keeping a healthy amount of potassium in your body. If they're not working right, you may get too much or too little.

If you have too much potassium in your blood, it can cause cardiac arrest -- when your heart suddenly stops beating.

If you have too little potassium in your blood, it can cause an irregular heartbeat. Your muscles may also feel weak."

Hang on, here's the last P – phosphorous. That's the one element you usually don't find on food labels. For CKD patients, that's pretty annoying since you may have to keep track of all 3 Ps and 1S at your nephrologist's or renal dietitian's direction. Mayo Clinic, another trusted site I've been consulting for over a dozen years, explains:

"Phosphorus is a mineral that's found naturally in many foods and also added to many processed foods. When you eat foods that have phosphorus in them, most of the phosphorus goes into your blood. Healthy kidneys remove extra phosphorus from the blood.

If your kidneys don't work well, you can develop a high phosphorus level in your blood, putting you at greater risk of heart disease, weak bones, joint pain and even death ....

How much phosphorus you need depends on your kidney function. If you have early-stage kidney disease or you're on dialysis, you may need to limit phosphorus. Nearly every food contains some phosphorus, so this can be hard to do."

While National Nutrition Month is for everyone, we – as CKD patients – need to pay more than usual attention to our nutrition if we don't want our chronic kidney disease to go spiraling out of control. Naturally, our diets need to be individualized based on the stage of our disease and diet is not all there is to slowing down the progression of the decline of your kidney function (the definition of CKD), but it's a start.

3/21 *What's the Supply Chain Got to Do with Us?*

That's a good question. As a chronic kidney patient stage 3b, it hasn't got too much to do with me except for which foods are available. As a diabetic, I may have trouble getting insulin down the line… and I don't mean due to the price. But some of my readers on dialysis are having problems right now due to the supply chain.

When I first heard the term 'supply chain,' I took guesses as to what it might mean. Let me spare you from that. The phrase wasn't included in my favorite dictionary, the **Merriam-Webster**, so I turned to Dictionary.com:

"marketing a channel of distribution beginning with the supplier of materials or components, extending through a manufacturing process to the distributor and retailer, and ultimately to the consumer"

In this case, the consumer is the dialysis patient with the retailer being the dialysis clinic. The distributor is probably the representative of the manufacturing company. The shortage I've been reading about is that of dialysate. But what is that?

This time my favorite dictionary came through:

"the material that passes through the membrane in dialysis"

As a non-dialysis CKD patient, my first question was "What membrane?" Luckily, the National Center for Biotechnology Institute [NCBI] explained simply:

"The blood and dialysis fluid are separated only by a thin wall, called a semipermeable membrane. This membrane allows particles that the body needs to get rid of to pass through it, but doesn't let important parts of the blood (e.g. blood cells) pass through."

Okay now, back to our original quest to figure out how the supply chain is affecting dialysis patients.

Take a look at these quotes on KHOU [Houston, Texas] in late January of this year:

"Statement of Brad Puffer, spokesperson for Fresenius Medical Care North America:

'We recognize the critical need for these supplies for patients requiring dialysis treatment. Our delivery drivers and manufacturing employees have been impacted by the latest wave of COVID-19 which has resulted in regional delivery and supply challenges. This has occurred despite a high vaccination rate among our employees and strict safety procedures in place.

'We are committed to resolving this unprecedented situation and have gone to great lengths to deliver dialysis supplies, including bringing in volunteer employees from other parts of the company and National Guard members to supplement our workforce. Our company will continue to work tirelessly to resolve these issues in order to maintain high-quality patient care.'

Statement of Dr. Jeffrey Hymes, Chief Medical Officer for Fresenius Kidney Care:

'In emergency situations, it is sometimes necessary to temporarily adjust the dialysis prescription to optimally utilize available resources. These decisions are made at the direction of our patients' treating physicians with attention to the needs of each individual. We know from our previous experience in natural disasters that these changes can be made while still meeting the standards for adequate dialysis. Our patients' health and safety remain our top priority.'"

So, it's not that there's a dearth of dialysate, but that Covid has caused a need for more and also knocked out many of the necessary workers. Covid is a pandemic [worldwide illness], which may become endemic [common illness]. If dialysis patients' time on the machine that saves their lives is shortened, how safe will they be?

MyHealth.Alberta.ca answers that question:

"If you don't get enough dialysis treatment, you may have extra fluid that stays in your body and causes swelling you'll see in your legs and arms. This is called fluid overload. Your blood also holds on to more of your body's waste products, making it more likely that you'll feel sick. Too much of your body's waste products in your blood is called uremia.

Uremia and fluid overload can cause:

you to feel weak and tired all the time

shortness of breath

high blood pressure between dialysis treatments

blood pressure to go down or drop during dialysis

inflammation of the heart muscle (swelling, redness, soreness)

higher risk for infection

problems with bleeding

poor appetite, nausea, and real weight loss

inability to tolerate exercise

a bitter taste in your mouth

yellow skin

itchy skin"

These are not exactly unprecedented times since there was the pandemic of 1918, but dialysis was not invented until the 1940s, so that's not a lot of help.

There are two types of dialysis. WebMD defines them:

"Hemodialysis: Your blood is put through a filter outside your body, cleaned, and then returned to you. This is done either at a dialysis facility or at home.

Peritoneal dialysis: Your blood is cleaned inside your body. A special fluid is put into your abdomen to absorb waste from the blood that passes through small vessels in your abdominal cavity. The fluid is then drained away. This type of dialysis is typically done at home."

Guess what cleans your blood. That's right, dialysate. Does this mean you're doomed if you're on dialysis? Is this a blog of gloom and doom? No, not at all. In late February of this year, ABC 2 News in Baltimore shared the following:

"A DaVita spokesperson wrote:

'Given the urgency of the situation, patients' physicians temporarily adjusted prescriptions as we concurrently notified patients—both in person and in writing. These adjustments ordered by our patients' physicians are backed by research and proven safe and effective.'

The National Kidney Foundation said treatments can safely be adjusted if patients are closely monitored.

'I would consider this approach as contingency management to avoid needing to go to crisis management,' wrote Dr. Pavlesky."

Rest assured. You are being well taken care of.

3/28 *Another New (to me) Kidney Disease*

It amazes me that after writing this blog for over a dozen years, I can still happen across something about the kidneys that I didn't know. This week it's Acute Tubular Necrosis. Have you ever heard of this before?

Way back in 2010, I defined acute in ***What Is It and How Did I Get It? Early Stage Kidney Disease:***

"**Acute:** Extremely painful, severe, or serious, quick onset, of short duration; the opposite of chronic."

I'm going to go back even further back to my college textbook, ***Latin & Greek in Current Use, Second Edition***, for the definition of necrosis:

"corpse"

Or, updated for our purposes, dead.

I think we can handle tubular with my favorite dictionary, ***the Merriam-Webster Dictionary***:

"having the form of or consisting of a tube. made or provided with tubes."

Putting it all together, it's the sudden onset of dead tubes. It can't be that simplistic and this definition doesn't make that much sense. So, I went to Medline for a more comprehensive definition:

"Acute tubular necrosis (ATN) is a kidney disorder involving damage to the tubule cells of the kidneys, which can lead to acute kidney failure. The tubules are tiny ducts in the kidneys that help filter the blood when it passes through the kidneys.

Got it. Well, what can cause ATN? The Cleveland Clinic was helpful here:

"The most frequent causes of acute tubular necrosis are a stroke or a heart attack, conditions that reduce oxygen to the kidneys.

Chemicals can also damage the tubules. These include X-ray contrast dye, anesthesia drugs, antibiotics and other toxic chemicals."

That's one of the reasons cardiology and nephrology are so connected. Avoid cardiology problems and you're helping yourself to avoid ATN. One of the three kinds of stroke is hemorrhagic. It's caused by a burst or blockage of blood vessels in your brain and can be affected by any blood vessel problem. One of the causes of hemorrhagic stroke is high blood pressure which just happens to be one of the causes of chronic kidney disease. It's also logical; if your blood can't reach your kidneys due to the blockage, your kidneys will be damaged.

Well, how do you know if you have ATN? Healthline lists the symptoms for us:

"The symptoms of ATN vary depending on its severity. You may:

feel drowsy even during the day

feel lethargic or physically drained

be excessively thirsty or experience dehydration

urinate very little or not at all

retain fluid or experience swelling in your body

have episodes of confusion

experience nausea or vomiting"

I'm glad I stumbled across ATN. It sounds like something important all CKD patients should know about. By the way, do you see a cardiologist? Speak with your nephrologist to see if it's something they'd recommend.

We know what ATN is, what causes it, and what the symptoms are, but what do you do about it if find you have ATN?

Wait. I have to share this with you. It's Medscape's information about ATN that we haven't come across yet:

"Acute tubular necrosis (ATN) is the most common cause of acute kidney injury (AKI) in the renal category (that is, AKI in which the pathology lies within the kidney itself). The term ATN is actually a misnomer, as there is minimal cell necrosis and the damage is not limited to tubules."

That sounds worse! We'd better get on to what to do about ATN if you find you have it. WebMD had quite a bit of information about treatment:

"The exact treatment that your doctor recommends will depend on the cause of your acute tubular necrosis.

If your acute tubular necrosis is caused by some form of poisoning, the most important treatment will be clearing the harmful substance out of your body. Then, you need to make sure that you know how the poison got into your body so it doesn't happen again.

Normally, your kidneys will be able to heal on their own. This means that your treatment will be focused on preventing the buildup of fluids and waste products in your body.

Your treatment phase can last anywhere from a few days to over six weeks. It depends on how badly damaged your kidneys are. Treatment methods can include:

Dialysis. In some cases, your doctor may decide that you need dialysis, a process that removes waste, salt, and fluids to prevent them from building up in the body while your kidneys are healing. They'll decide this on a case-by-case basis.

Dietary changes. Sometimes, you'll also need to change your diet during your recovery. Helpful changes could include limiting how much fluid and sodium you eat and drink. This way, you don't add to the fluid build-up that's caused by the acute tubular necrosis.

Medications. In some cases, your doctor will prescribe medications to take during your recovery. These include ones to help increase how often you urinate or to control potassium levels in your body.

If this condition is left untreated, your kidneys could fail. This could mean that you need to make life-long changes to manage the symptoms from the tissue damage."

The Merck Manual (Consumer Version) offers us both good and bad news:

"Outcome depends on correction of the disorder that caused acute tubular necrosis. If that disorder responds rapidly to treatment, kidney function usually returns to normal in 1 to 3 weeks. Prognosis is usually better if people's urine volume exceeds 400 mL (about 13.5 ounces) every 24 hours. People who are more seriously ill, especially those who require care in an intensive care unit, have a higher risk of death."

There's another reason to take extra good care of both your heart and your kidney health. Should you end up with ATN, you want to be one of those "otherwise healthy patients." It all sounds bad but be careful rather than afraid.

4/4 *Does Coffee Count?*

We all have water guidelines. Those on dialysis need to keep it down and those who aren't need to keep it up. For example, my nephrologist suggested 64 ounces per day. That's the equivalent of eight glasses of eight ounces each. To be honest, I use a water bottle that has the ounces marked on it. It's just easier.

Yet, eight ounces is not right for everyone. The National Kidney Foundation makes several recommendations: men usually need about 13 ounces while women need nine; and using their own words:

"A common misconception is that everyone should drink eight glasses of water per day, but since everyone is different, daily water needs will vary by person. How much water you need is based on differences in age, climate, exercise intensity, as well as states of pregnancy, breastfeeding, and illness."

Umm, why do we need water anyway? The Southeastern Massachusetts Dialysis Group tells us as chronic kidney disease patients [pre-dialysis also despite the group's name],

"Water helps your kidneys remove waste from your blood. Your body excretes these wastes and excess fluids in the form of urine that travels to your bladder before leaving your body. Water also helps keep your arteries open so that your blood can flow freely to your kidneys. This blood delivers oxygen and nutrients that help your kidneys function. Dehydration makes it more difficult for this delivery system to work.

Mild dehydration can impair normal bodily functions, including your kidneys. Severe dehydration can actually lead to kidney damage. Drinking fluids is the best way to avoid dehydration, especially when you work or exercise especially hard or in warm or humid weather.

People with diabetes, kidney disease or other illnesses that affect the kidneys need to take in adequate amounts of fluid to keep their kidneys performing well. People with low blood pressure need to take in plenty of fluids to maintain kidney health, for example. Your kidneys act like filters to remove toxins from your body. To push blood through the filters, though, the blood has to be moving with force; in cases of low blood pressure, there is not enough pressure to force the blood through the tiny filters of the kidneys."

Notice, please that the word 'water' has been replaced by the word 'fluid.'

But wait a minute, I drink two eight-ounce cups of black coffee most every day. Coffee is mostly water, isn't it? Does that count in my water – or fluid – allowance? Let's figure it out. I went to Everyday Health for this information:

"There are so many different types of coffee to choose from, and your personal preference will affect how much hydration you'll get from your brew. Two main factors dictate how much hydration you'll be getting: the amount of caffeine and the volume of the beverage. For example, according to Mayo Clinic, an 8-oz cup of regular brewed coffee contains about 96 mg of caffeine while the same sized cup of decaffeinated brewed coffee contains only 2 mg of caffeine. This means, while you'll be getting about 7 oz of hydration from the regular coffee, you'll be getting the full 8 oz of fluid from the decaf. Caffeinated instant coffee falls somewhere in between, with 62 mg of caffeine per 8-oz serving. Similarly, a 1-oz serving of espresso contains about 64 mg of caffeine, which gives it almost as much diuretic power as a full 8 oz of caffeinated coffee, but since that's all packed into only 1 oz of fluid, you're really not getting any hydration from a shot of espresso."

Wow! That means I'm getting 14 of my 64 ounces from my favorite beverage. I only drink water and the black coffee, but if I'm ill or having stomach problems, I will eat soup. Is that a fluid, too?

My favorite dictionary, the Merriam-Webster, defines soup for us:

"a liquid food especially with a meat, fish, or vegetable stock as a base and often containing pieces of solid food"

Double wow! So even if I'm not that hungry and just have a cup of soup, there's another eight ounces or so of liquid, or as I see it being called now, hydration. So now I've had about 24 of my 64 ounces of liquid [no longer just water and sometimes called hydration] requirement for the day.

Hmmm, if soup counts as a liquid and coffee counts as a liquid [tea, too], what else does? Thanks to the American Kidney Fund's Kidney Kitchen for the following:

"Examples of fluid:

Ice

Soups and stews

Pudding

Ice cream, sherbet, sorbet, popsicles, etc.

Protein drinks (Nepro, Novasource, Ensure, etc.)

All beverages (water, soda, tea, coffee, milk, nondairy milk, etc.)

Jell-O® other gelatin products and gelatin substitutes (pectin, arrowroot powder, etc.)"

Triple wow! So, if you get tired of water, water, water [I don't.] to fulfill your fluid or hydration needs, look at the variety of foods you can have. Of course, if you have diabetes, you'd have to get the sugar free versions of these foods… and, please, no chemical artificial sweeteners. Sort of opens up the world of fluids, doesn't it? [Notice I'm using the word 'fluids' or the word 'hydration' instead of the word 'water."]

St. Joseph's Healthcare, Hamilton has a bit more information for us:

"Fluid is a liquid or any food that turns into a liquid at room temperature…. Fruits and vegetables naturally contain water. If consumed in moderation, fruits and vegetables should not contribute large volumes of water to your daily total intake of fluids. Therefore, fruits and vegetables do not need to be counted as part of your daily fluid intake."

I prefer to stick with my water and coffee but look at all the foods that have been made available to you. My favorite treat as a child was chocolate pudding. I remember the smooth, rich creaminess of it. My brother's was orange jello. He said it felt cool going down his throat. I'll be content with my memories. You go enjoy these foods.

4/11 *But How Do I Remember?*

It's common knowledge that our kidneys love water [unless you're on dialysis]. It's also common knowledge that many of us have problems combining the kidney and diabetic diets. In the United States, under Medicare you're entitled to two hours of a dietician's time per year if you have chronic kidney disease. Well, three the first year of your diagnosis. If you're not on Medicare, you'd have to check your insurance. Many of them do cover dieticians.

I took advantage of Medicare's offering and am seeing a dietitian in order to combine the kidney and diabetic diets. Actually, I'm seeing him virtually. We had a zoom visit yesterday and somehow got on the topic of how to remember to drink the amount of water I need daily. I thought I'd set a reminder on my phone for every hour, but then he reminded me there are apps that will alert you to drink water.

Naturally, that got me to thinking about these apps… and feeling sure we could all use whatever information I found about them. Ladies and gentlemen, prepare to hydrate.

Although I wanted the app for my iPhone or Apple Watch, I used my computer to search. My first search was for 'best free hydration reminder apps for 2022.' Waterllama caught my eye, not just for the cute name, but for its 4.9 out of 5 star rating. This app does offer in app upgrades, although the basic app is free. According to their website,

"… • Smart drink water reminders during your day

• Track water in any drink: water, tea, matcha, coffee, juice, smoothie, soup, soda, beer, wine, cider, vermouth, liquor, etc [sic]

- Fun Challenges: Sober Bear, Weight Loss Sloth, No Cheat Cheetah
- Widget
- Streaks habit tracker free
- Fill up cute characters
- Celebrate your day with a shareable recap illustration
- Calculate daily water intake goal based on your weight, activity & weather
- Set Custom drinking water goal
- Custom drinks - set a name, icon, cup size, hydration ratio & caffeine
- Water intake calendar
- Apple Health sync
- Oz/Ml units
- Water tracker Apple Watch app....
- Waterllama now remembers your last 3 intake amounts for any beverage that you add on a daily basis. You can quickly swipe or tap through them and add instantly without interacting with the cup.
- You can also tap the dots icon at the bottom right of the screen to enter the exact amount manually."

Although the app is from the Ukraine, they are up and running despite Russia's invading their country.

My Water – Daily Water Tracker is rated 4.8 out of 5 stars, but there isn't much information on their site.

"It helps and motivates you to drink water according to the schedule and will keep the water drinking logs, including the quantity and time you drink water....

This app has been updated by Apple to display the Apple Watch app icon."

What's nice about this app is that up to six members of the family can share it and it's also available for your iPad.

Despite its 4.2 star rating, Daily Water-Drink Reminder is the one I chose for myself. The description from their website will explain why:

"- Set goal amount of daily drinking water and track it.

- Log amount of daily drinking water.

- Touch to log each drinking.

- Check glasses of water drunk each day.

- Customize volume of each glass of water.

- Customize how much of water you drink each time, 1/4 glass, 1/2 glass or A glass.

- Plan drinking schedule and it will remind you when it's time.

- 10 free alert sounds to choose.

- Histogram to show the amount of your one day's, recent one week's and one month's amount of drinking water.

- Show amount of glasses of water you have drunk one day on the icon.

- Email the data of date, amount of water to anyone you would like.

- Supports transferring data to Health app.

- Supports WiFi backup & restore.

- Supports Dropbox backup and restore.

- Support oz and ml.

- Supports Apple Watch version.

- Supports 3D Touch function.

- Supports Today Widget."

What especially drew me was the simple entering of how much you drank on each of the water glasses in the app. Simple is the way I like to go.

I'm sure by now, Android users are starting to feel left out. Don't. Another 4.5 rated app, Water Drink Reminder - Hydro is one of those for you:

"★ Water demand calculator – will calculate and suggest the amount of water to drink each day
★ Reminders – will ensure regular hydration
★ Charts and statistics - will show your progress as you regularly drink water
★ Adjustable sizes of containers - adjust them to your needs
★ Multilanguage （Deutsch, English, Español, Français, Italiano, Русский, Polski, Português, 中文, 日本語）
★ automatic backup copies in a cloud
★ data transfer between various devices
★ access to analyses and charts from web browser (http://hydro-app.com)"

Another Android app, with a 4.8 rating this time, is Water Drink Reminder. This is from their website:

" * Water tracker that will remind you when and how much water to drink throughout the day
  * Customized cup and standard (oz) or metric (ml) units
  * You can set your start and end time to drink water for each day
  * Graph and logs of your schedule
  * Syncs weight data with Google Fit.
  * Syncs weight and drink water data with S Health.
  * You can login through your Google account.
  * You can backup and restore your drinking data through the water tracker."

As you can see, there are slight differences among the features the apps offer. This is all new to me and slightly overwhelming. That's why I thought if I started you off in your search, it may not be overwhelming to you. Let's remember I'm not the expert here.

4/18 *Leftovers*

The last time Easter, Passover, and Ramadan coincided was 33 years ago. This year, Passover started on the evening of April 15, Easter Sunday – the end of Holy Week – fell on either April 17 (for Western Christendom) or will fall on April 24 (for Eastern Orthodoxy), and the month-long fast of Ramadan began on April 2. That's a lot of special food for the kidney diet.

True, most of these holidays are over, but what to do with the leftover special food? Let's take a look. I'll start with Passover food since that's what I'm most familiar with. First thing you should know is that Jews do not eat leavened bread, only matzoh which is unleavened, during the seven or eight days of Passover. That symbolizes that the Jews needed to leave Egypt quickly, so quickly that there wasn't time for their bread to rise.

My mother made terrific matzoh ball soup... and she made a lot of it. Enough so there would be plenty left over for us to store in the refrigerator and send some home with guests. You can do the same providing it's low sodium. After all, it's just chicken stock, carrots, celery, and matzoh balls, although you may make it a little differently. Did you know that low sodium matzoh ball mix is readily available?

The main course for Passover in my home was baked chicken and roasted vegetables. This is so easy. If you've cooked with no sodium spices instead of salt, all you need to do is warm up the leftovers. No wonder my mother made so much. She didn't have to cook for the rest of the week!

When I started hosting the seders as an adult, I did the same thing. Once I was diagnosed with chronic kidney disease, I found myself surprised at how little change I had to make to this meal to ensure it was kidney friendly. All I had to do was keep it low sodium. Sometimes, the warmed-up leftovers even tasted better than when they were originally served.

Easter celebrates the resurrection of Jesus for Christians. I've made one or two Easter meals for my husband, stepdaughters, and sons-in-law. This was a little more difficult because it was a meat meal. They preferred a standing rib roast. I'm not much of a red meat eater so I had to ask the butcher what it looked like and then I needed to look up recipes. Despite how many of us were at these Easter dinners, there were leftovers. You guessed it, having used sodium free spices in the cooking, all I had to do was warm up the leftovers. Well, that's not exactly true, just as with the Passover meal, I had to be careful about how much of the chicken for that meal or the standing rib roast for this one I had. Everyone's different, but my nephrologist keeps me capped at five ounces of protein per day.

We had served only kidney friendly vegetables with this but had no leftovers. So, we made a fresh salad with carrots, a few mushrooms, and just a bit of spinach to go with the standing roast leftovers. Simple, tasty, and kidney friendly. We used few mushrooms and spinach because they are high in potassium, one of the things CKD patients need to be aware of.

Come to think of it, the only problem with the leftovers for both Passover and Easter were the desserts. DaVita has a tasty recipe for Apple Cinnamon Farfel Kugel for Passover. They also have a mouthwatering recipe for Strawberry Pie for Easter. I'm offering you these suggestions because I usually don't deal with dessert, serving fresh fruit and coffee instead. I do acknowledge that dessert is the crowning glory of meals, especially holiday meals, for some people whether they are CKD patients or not. The Peeps and chocolates my kids brought to the meal offer proof of that statement.

Now to tackle a Ramadan meal. First, you need to know that Muslims fast from dawn to dusk each of the one-month days of Ramadan. That means the meals are extra special. There are many recipes for the before dawn meal, but scrambled eggs seem to be the quickest and easiest. Yes, you can make enough to have leftovers. You just need to remember to spice it with no sodium spices (think something like Mrs. Dash spices.) and watch your protein limit.

Breaking the fast after dusk requires something an empty stomach can handle. One such food is Rice Roti, as Americans call it. You may already be aware of the ingredients: water, oil, rice flour. [This is a good recipe for me since I have a wheat sensitivity.] You may know it as Tandal Achi Bhakri or Pathiri. It's low potassium and saltless the way CKD patients make it. Be careful of the accompaniments you choose. You are watching your sodium, potassium, phosphorous, and protein intake, right? It's usually cooked on a tava or cooking pan. You may know it as a sac or saj. You can use a frying pan instead if you'd rather.

Okay, so what do you do with the leftovers? Since they are already salt and potassium free, you simply warm them up and add the accompaniments. One could be cranberry dip with fresh fruit, providing you don't have hyperkalemia [high potassium]. Another might be corn idlis. DaVita has some good recipes with electrolyte counts included. Oh, but we're talking about leftovers, aren't we? Again, heat or chill your accompaniments as needed.

The one thing to be careful about is the desserts. Many are made with dried fruits. These are extremely high in potassium since potassium becomes concentrated in such foods.

Maybe living life on the kidney diet is not as hard as we may have thought. Leftovers certainly are easy if the food is cooked according to the kidney diet in the first place. As for cooking – even special holiday foods – there are numerous websites and cookbooks to help. Hmmm, maybe that should be the topic of next week's blog.

4/25 *Surprise!*

Last week, I mentioned that this week's blog would be about chronic kidney disease cookbooks and food preparation blogs. That's what I'd planned at the time. But then a guest blog appeared in my mailbox.

Lori Hartwell, the author, is one of the first people I met when I decided I wanted to become a CKD awareness advocate. She was kind enough to publish several of my articles. Recently, we met again since we were both working on the same zoom project. We talked about swapping guest blogs… and then life got in the way, as it usually does. Being a person of her word, she didn't forget. I'll turn this blog over to Lori now.

*****

Kidney Disease Diagnosis: Help is Out There

By Lori Hartwell

I've lived with kidney disease since the age of 2, back when the medical world was first learning how to treat the disease. I was not expected to live. Dialysis was in its infancy stages back in 1968, and so was I. The medical community became my world. I earned my education as a patient, while spending so much of my time in hospitals and in being the first to try a new treatment. It was a lonely start in life as I missed many childhood experiences. I spent all my teenager years on dialysis.

Years later, after beating all odds, I started the Renal Support Network (RSN). I did it because I didn't want others with kidney disease to feel as lonely as I once did. I wanted to let them know if they become knowledgeable about their illness, proactive in their care they will realize there is lots of hope!

In 1993 I started RSN as a support network for others, like myself, who live with chronic kidney disease. Peer support is important to learn how to deal with all the emotions and to navigate this illness – "One friend can make the difference." We have expanded our programs to help people have hope and to be proactive in their care.

As RSN's President and Founder, it is my goal to give people living with chronic kidney disease (CKD) tools to take control of the course and management of this life-threatening illness. It's hard to believe through our patient engagement programs we have grown to reach millions of people.

It is important to be aware of the epidemic of kidney disease. The Center for Disease Control states that more than 15% of the adult population in the United States live with chronic kidney disease (CKD). It's possible to have kidney disease and not know. Don't be afraid to get tested. Kidney function can be maintained, and the progression of the disease can be slowed down if caught in the early stages. Don't be afraid to get tested it is a simple blood test. An ounce of prevention is worth a pound of cure.

It is also believed that people with CKD tend to have higher levels of anxiety and depression than others. They often feel isolated because of their outward appearances which make them different than their peers. They also have different priorities in life. When others are thinking about "the big game" or which nail salon offers the best manicure, people with CKD are struggling to understand the disease and learn how to live a full life despite the fact that they have CKD.

Help is out there! Having even one friend can really make a difference. Connect with the Renal Support Network where you'll find a variety of national, online patient support group activities to curb the loneliness that so often affects those with CKD. Chances are you'll find more than one friend if you make that connection. And always be careful about depression. It can sneak up on you! Read the book, "Chronically Happy – Joyful Living in Spite of Chronic Illness," and be inspired. It is my personal story of deciding to take simple, logical steps to live a full life and realize one's dreams.

Perhaps you are having difficulty understanding kidney disease. Knowledge is power! Listen in to the Essentials of Chronic Kidney Disease podcast to hear Dr. Stephen Fadem, a nephrologist in Houston, Texas, speak as he sheds light on CKD. He talks about the steps you can take in collaboration with your physician to either delay the progression of your disease or, in many instances, prevent it. Many people are not even aware that they have CKD, so be sure to be tested during your annual physical. Worried about your diet? The CKD Diet – What to Know Based on New Science by Dr. Kam Kalantar will be helpful.

Learning can be fun, and you'll see how when you check out the animated video, "Share Your Spare." You'll be introduced to Neff and Nuff, the two "kidney pals" who talk about what it means to donate the "gift of life." If you share the video with your friends and family, it may encourage them to register to become organ donors. Watch the entire animated series on our website.

Or maybe you are one of the many people living with CKD who need help with your diet. If so, this podcast, the "What's for Dinner" blues, is for you! There's been talk about low-protein diets, but keep in mind that your body still needs a certain amount of protein. Adding more plant-based sources of protein may help. It's important to talk to a renal dietitian to know what is right for you.

I have seen the evolution of this illness for 50 plus years of living kidney disease. Although living with CKD can be difficult, the illness is manageable, especially when you have the opportunity to learn from other people's experiences and wisdom, so make connections!

Visit https://www.rsnhope.org/ today, join us and hang onto hope!

5/2 **Food!**

This was meant to be last week's blog... until Lori Hartwell of RSNHope gifted us with a guest blog, that is. No way I was going to pass that goody up. Since I'm the scheduler as well as the writer, it was easy to change what would be posted when. But a promise is a promise. So, today we talk about chronic kidney disease cookbooks and food preparation sites.

What better place to start than the *National Kidney Foundation*? They make life easy by dividing their information into different categories. This is from their website:

"Kidney disease stages 1-4
How a healthy diet to [sic] help prevent the progression of kidney disease.

Dialysis
Most patients on dialysis need to limit the amount of sodium, potassium, and phosphorus in their diets.

Transplant
After a kidney transplant, your diet will still be an important part of maintaining your overall health.

Kidney Stones

If you have had kidney stones, you may need to follow a special diet to prevent kidney stones coming back."

Not only do you find different diets and reasons for eating that way for each condition, but there is a 'find a renal dietitian' link. You can also enter a search for recipes by using the search function in the upper right-hand corner of any of their pages.

How about the American Kidney Foundation? Have you tried their Kidney Kitchen yet? They had 657 CKD friendly recipes at last count. If you click 'Find Recipes' on their home page, this is what will pop up:

"Difficulty Levels   Nutrients   Meal Types   Dietary Requirements   Collection"

Each of these has a detailed dropdown menu. For example, should you choose 'Meal Types,' you'd have a choice of 'Lunch, Dinner, Sides, Breakfast, Dessert, Snacks, Drinks, or Condiments.' Now that's convenient.

The American Association of Kidney Patients (AAKP) has some delicious menus you can download. For instance,

"Overnight Oats

No-Crust Quiche with Leeks

Basmati Summer Salad

Zesty Chickpea Stew

Hamburger New Style

Pineapple Beef Stir-fry

Garlic Shrimp Linguini

Summer Chicken Breast

Fine Fish Stew

Pear and Ginger Upside Down Cake

Dutch Apple Soufflé

Tropical Mocktail"

These recipes are from their **AAKP Delicious! sixth edition.** You can order recipe cards and even some select issues of earlier **AAKP Delicious!** editions.

I see that dialysis centers such as DaVita and Fresenius have recipes available for those on dialysis. DaVita even has downloadable cookbooks, while Fresenius has 320 downloadable recipes. I must say my mouth is starting to water from reading all these luscious recipes.

Let's take a look at hold-in-your-hands cookbooks for those who are not interested in downloading and/or printing recipes. My favorite is still **Renal Diet Cookbook for the Newly Diagnosed: The Complete Guide to Managing Kidney Disease and Avoiding Dialysis** by Susan Zogheib MHS RD LDN, probably for her meatballs alone. Although we did enjoy the other recipes we tried from this book. This is the book description on Amazon:

"Your new kidney-friendly diet made easy with meal plans and flavorful recipes

When you've just been diagnosed with stage 1-4 chronic kidney disease, learning to follow diet restrictions can be a challenge. But your meals don't have to be complicated or boring to support your health and slow the disease's progression. Keep it simple and flavorful with the **Renal Diet Cookbook for the Newly Diagnosed**. This practical cookbook equips you with essential info, 4 weekly meal plans, and 100 easy, kidney-healthy recipes to kick-start your renal diet.

Find out how kidney disease works, and learn how diet plays a key role in keeping you healthy and avoiding dialysis. Explore at-a-glance food charts to help you regulate nutrients like sodium, potassium, phosphorus, and protein. All of the book's recipes include nutrition facts, and many can be made in 30 minutes or less—accommodating your busy schedule and helping keep your kidney-friendly diet stress-free.

The Renal Diet Cookbook for the Newly Diagnosed includes:

100+ Satisfying recipes—Enjoy Buckwheat Pancakes, Creamy Broccoli Soup, Lemon Garlic Halibut, Meatloaf with Mushroom Gravy, Strawberry Pie, and much more.

4 Weekly meal plans—Get started with four weeks of daily menus, complete with shopping lists, snack suggestions, and nutrition facts for every recipe.

5 Steps to a renal diet—Take your new diet one step at a time in five practical stages, including specific guidance for reading food labels and controlling portions."

I thought a more well-known author might appeal to those of you who like already having heard about the author:

"The Cooking Doc's Kidney-Healthy Cooking: A Modern 10-Step Guide to Preventing and Managing Kidney Disease by Dr. Blake Shusterman

Dr. Blake Shusterman is a board certified nephrologist (kidney doctor) and creator of the YouTube cooking show 'The Cooking Doc.'

In this book he combines his medical knowledge, real world patient care experience and his passion for delicious food to create an easy to follow 10-step guide for preventing and managing kidney disease and a collection of meticulously tested recipes that are accessible and home cook friendly.

If you or your family members are searching for the best dietary recommendations to manage and prevent kidney disease, this book can help set you on the right path no matter where you are in your journey. A combination of concrete health tips, scientific knowledge, inspirational stories, charts, and beautiful recipes and pictures, this book can help you understand the dietary needs for each stage of kidney disease and make you a better cook. From tweaked classics, such as Vegan Bolognese and Macaroni & Cheese, to modern and diverse fare such as Thai Shrimp Salad and Chicken Farro bowls, this book gives you more than 50 flavor packed, low sodium recipes alongside expert nutritional analysis, pro-tip sidebars, and cooking tips and techniques.

The 10-steps:

1. Understand Your Kidneys

2. Choose Your Beverages Wisely

3. Uncover Hidden Salt and #ChangeYourBuds

4. Embrace Plant-Based Eating

5. Get Potassium Right

6. Avoid High Protein Pitfalls

7. Discover Alkaline-Rich Foods

8. Identify and Eliminate Sneaky Phosphorus

9. Integrate the DASH, Mediterranean and Diabetic Diets into your Routine

10. Keep an Open Mind if you Start Dialysis

It must be lunchtime by now. I'm eager to get in the kitchen with all these recipe sources.

5/9 Chronic Kidney Disease Changed My Life

Those of us with CKD always say that, don't we? There's so much we have to change about our lives once we're diagnosed. That is, if you want to keep your CKD under control and possibly slow down its progression. There are the dietary changes to start. Then the medications. Don't forget the lifestyle changes: exercise, avoid alcohol, no drinking, rest, adequate sleep. We all know the drill.

However, those are not the only things that changed in my life. I'd written 'how to's, literary guides, and study guides for decades. I'd taught research writing on the college level… and I'd earned an Academic Certificate in Creative Writing. Add my having been a teacher for most of my adult life and you have the basis for a CKD awareness advocate. That is how my life changed the most with my diagnosis.

The first thing I did was research for myself. I then decided that was pretty selfish. What about the people who didn't understand what their nephrologists were saying and didn't know how to research for themselves? Keep in mind, this was back in 2008 way before the patient based treatment movement began.

I had never published a book myself. Rather, I had always written for publishers at their request. That changed with my desire to become an advocate for CKD awareness. My thinking was, "Who's going to publish a book about CKD for patients by a lay person?" I was and I did. **What Is It and How Did I Get it? Early Stage Chronic Kidney Disease** was the first book. I kept it reader friendly and explained what I hadn't understood and what others had asked me about.

That sparked a bunch of readings at bookstores, coffee shops, and civic clubs. Then the book was mentioned in various publications, both locally and nationally. I was getting the word out! The book and its information also ignited requests from various groups for articles and/or caused those groups I'd requested to write for to change their minds and say yes. I even organized a Kidney Walk out here in Arizona. And now I serve as a patient advisor for two pharmaceutical companies.

What struck me the most was when an Indian doctor told me about how very poor his patients were and that he wanted them to have the information in the book, but they couldn't possibly afford it.

Together, we worked out a plan for me to blog a chapter a week. He would print each week's blog and make multiple copies for his patients. Great! Now I just needed to learn how to blog.

Again, I did... with the help of my older daughter. Thank goodness she knew what she was doing because I didn't. But it worked. I blogged as **SlowItDownCKD**. Once the books' chapters were all blogged, I was having such fun being a CKD awareness advocate that I didn't want to stop. So, I didn't and that's where the **SlowItDownCKD** book series began. Each year I would gather that year's blogs and format them into a book. At this point, they go from 2011 to 2021.

You're right; no one can keep covering the basics of CKD for a decade. I branched out into writing about dialysis, transplant, pediatric nephrology, and different kinds of kidney disease. There were also guest blogs from the adult children of CKD patients, transplantees, other CKD writers, and innovators.

I no longer give book talks or participate in meetings, unless they are online. Covid and cancer took my energy. But I still write and will continue to do so. I still feel it's important that people know about this disease. So many have CKD and don't know it. It's sort of sad since all it takes is a blood test and a urine test to be diagnosed. I urge you to keep telling your friends and family how easy it is to make certain they're not part of the club no one wants to join. Thanks for taking the time to read my story.

And thanks to all the readers who share the blog, talk to others about it, buy the books and share them with friends and family. Thanks to all those who urge their friends and family to get tested, who go with them to be tested, and who accompany them to be an extra ear at their nephrology appointments. And thanks to those who urge their nephrologists to remember to explain and ask questions of their patients.

According to the Centers for Disease Control and Prevention (CKD):

"**More than 1 in 7**, that is 15% of US adults or 37 million people, are estimated to have CKD. As many as 9 in 10 adults with CKD do not know they have CKD. About 2 in 5 adults with severe CKD do not know they have CKD."

That is as of last year and only for the United States. I turned to MedAlertHelp to find the global statistics:

"The global estimated CKD prevalence is between 11.7% and 15.1%. To be more specific, that's around 13.4%, or 850 million people suffering from chronic kidney disease worldwide, as per chronic kidney disease statistics worldwide for 2020…."

That was two years ago. Imagine what it is now. Surely, you can see the need for CKD awareness. You can help. Start talking about chronic kidney disease... please.

5/16 *How Pets Help*

We've all heard that pets relax us. My family was a cat family until we moved into a house. We had so many dogs in Staten Island while the girls were growing up that I'm not sure I can remember them all. Here in Arizona, it's only been my Sweet Ms. Bella – who instantly loved Bear – and Shiloh, our present big, fluffy, white dog.

I'm particularly interested in how our pets can help us with our chronic kidney disease. This all started when I wondered out loud what I should write about for this week's blog. Bear kiddingly called out, "Pets!" He was being silly, but I liked the idea. Let's see if we can figure this out.

Here's what the CDC has to say about having pets:

"There are many health benefits of owning a pet. They can increase opportunities to exercise, get outside, and socialize. Regular walking or playing with pets can decrease blood pressure, cholesterol levels, and triglyceride levels. Pets can help manage loneliness and depression by giving us companionship. Most households in the United States have at least one pet.

Studies have shown that the bond between people and their pets is linked to several health benefits, including:

- Decreased blood pressure, cholesterol levels, triglyceride levels, feelings of loneliness, anxiety, and symptoms of PTSD.
- Increased opportunities for exercise and outdoor activities; better cognitive function in older adults; and more opportunities to socialize"

Now, let's apply that to CKD patients. Hypertension, or high blood pressure, is the second most common cause of chronic kidney disease. I turned to the National Institute of Diabetes and Digestive and Kidney Diseases [NIDDK] to pinpoint exactly how hypertension affects your kidneys:

"High blood pressure can constrict and narrow the blood vessels, which eventually damages and weakens them throughout the body, including in the kidneys. The narrowing reduces blood flow.

If your kidneys' blood vessels are damaged, they may no longer work properly. When this happens, the kidneys are not able to remove all wastes and extra fluid from your body. Extra fluid in the blood vessels can raise your blood pressure even more, creating a dangerous cycle, and cause more damage leading to kidney failure."

Thank you, Shiloh, with helping to keep my blood vessels unconstricted.

What about high cholesterol levels? WebMD was able to help us out here:

"Cholesterol is a waxy substance. Your body makes it and uses it to build your cells. You also get it from many foods. But having too much cholesterol can lead to health problems....

High cholesterol can build up in arteries to increase your risk of a heart attack or stroke. It turns out that high cholesterol isn't good for your kidneys either."

Along with high cholesterol, high triglycerides are detrimental to your kidneys. These fats in your blood can lead to diabetes, which is the foremost cause of CKD. High triglycerides might also raise your creatinine level. You need to remember that you do need some triglyceride since they store unused calories. These are used by your body for energy. You just don't want high triglycerides.

I had no idea my dogs and cats were helping me control my CKD. By the way, other pets can also help. It doesn't have to be a dog or cat.

We know – fortunately or not – that exercise if important if you have CKD. This is something I explored in my first CKD book: **What Is It and How Did I Get It? Early Stage Chronic Kidney Disease**:

"I knew exercise was important to control my weight. It would also improve my blood pressure and lower my cholesterol and triglyceride s. The greater your triglycerides, the greater the risk of increasing your creatinine. There were other benefits, too, although you didn't have to have CKD to enjoy them: better sleep and improved muscle function and strength. But, as with everything else you do that might impinge upon your health, check with your doctor before you start exercising….

Keeping it simple, basically, there's a compound released by voluntary muscle contraction. It tells the body to repair itself and grow stronger. The idea is to start exercising slowly and then intensify your activity….

What I didn't know at the time is that your body becomes accustomed to a certain kind of exercise and then it isn't as effective anymore."

I can't walk Shiloh since she ends up walking me, but we play. We run back and forth down the length of the long central hallway in the house. I'm certain you can figure out how to get some exercise playing with your pet if you, too, cannot walk him.

As an older adult, I was interested in the "better cognitive function in older adults" benefit of having a pet. As a CKD patient, I wondered if it would have any effect on CKD brain fog. The National Center For Biotechnology Information [NCBI] succinctly tells us via their work that not nothings been proven about this yet:

"Exercise interventions are likely to be beneficial based on biological plausibility and pilot trial data."

Relaxation is also helpful if you have CKD. Stress needs to be avoided. Petting your pet or otherwise spending time with them is relaxing. Avoiding stress is one of the ways you could help delay the worsening of your chronic kidney disease.

I like to rub behind Shiloh's ears. She loves it and it relaxes me. I also like to brush her. She leans into the brush, and I baby talk to her. Both of us benefit from this form of relaxation. Bear likes to rub her belly. Again, they both love it... and I'll bet they're both benefiting from this.

Yes, I do think pets help in dealing with your CKD. Who couldn't use lowered blood pressure, cholesterol, triglycerides, and a chance at extra stress relief? Do you have a pet? IF not, would you consider getting one after reading this blog?

5/23 **Bad Water**

I found this on a slip of paper on my desk... in my handwriting. I wasn't sure if this was for my #1 New Release for Chemotherapy on Amazon **Cancer Dancer**. But that was published last week. Then again, maybe it was the sequel (or prequel) I was thinking about for my time travel romance **Portal in Time**. Wait, maybe it was for a **SlowItDownCKD** blog. I was flummoxed. I figured I wouldn't know unless I researched it. Sure enough, I got a hit: lead in the water and chronic kidney disease patients.

Let's go with that. We know our kidneys love water, although your nephrologist may call it hydration. Many of us have been urged to drink 64 ounces daily. Obviously, not those on dialysis whose fluid intake is restricted. I've written about the fact that other liquids – like coffee or tea and anything that can melt to liquid form – count towards those 64 ounces. We know that sodas are one of the liquids we are to avoid, especially dark sodas since they contain phosphorous.

On to that lead in the water. While this is harmful for anyone, I wondered why it is especially harmful to those with CKD. This is from a *Journal of the American Society of Nephrology* article published last year:

"'For individuals with heightened susceptibility to lead exposure, such as those with chronic kidney disease, there is no safe amount of lead contamination of drinking water,' says John Danziger at Beth Israel Deaconess Medical Center in Massachusetts.

Danziger and his colleagues analysed health information from 597,968 patients with chronic kidney disease in the US who started dialysis between 2005 and 2017, as well as official data on lead concentrations in city water systems in the five years leading up to their dialysis initiation.

The team found that those who lived in cities with detectable levels of lead in the water systems had significantly lower concentrations of the oxygen-transporting protein haemoglobin in their blood before starting dialysis and during the first month of the therapy than people who lived where lead wasn't detectable in the water. Lead is known to interfere with the ability of blood cells to produce haemoglobin, increasing the risk of anaemia.

Every 0.01 milligram per litre increase in lead concentration in the water was associated with a 0.02 gram per decilitre reduction in haemoglobin concentration in people's blood.

The trend was observed even at lead levels below the US Environmental Protection Agency's threshold of 0.015 milligrams per litre, which mandates regulatory action that can include public education, water treatment and lead service line replacement. 'More comprehensive surveillance of household water is critical,' says Danziger."

Looks like a couple of definitions are in order. Hemoglobin [American spelling]:

"Transports oxygen in the blood via red blood cells and give the red blood cells their color"

While anemia [American spelling] is:

"A blood disease in which the number of red blood cells decreases"

Both these definitions are from my first CKD book: ***What Is It and How Did I Get It? Early Stage Chronic Kidney Disease***. Although that book was published over a decade ago, the definitions haven't changed.

Dr. Danziger mentions elsewhere in the article that he is referring to individuals with advanced CKD. What makes that even worse is that these people, those on dialysis, are the ones that need to limit their fluid intake. Do you remember that water is considered the best fluid for CKD patients?

MedPageToday has more from Dr. Danziger's study:

"'Our findings suggest that for those with kidney disease, there is no safe amount of lead in drinking water,' the researchers wrote. 'While water has generally been considered a minor cause of lead toxicity, increased absorption and decreased excretion in those with kidney disease confer an exaggerated susceptibility.'

Children are at increased risk from lead exposure, and the complications of chronic kidney disease (CKD) confer similar susceptibility, the investigators explained. Metabolic conditions prevalent in CKD, such as hypocalcemia, iron deficiency, and malnutrition, increase the proportion of lead absorbed across the gastrointestinal tract. In addition, patients with CKD excrete lead less effectively, resulting in circulating levels that are much higher than in individuals with normal renal function.

In addition to its neurological, cardiovascular, and endocrine effects, lead can also cause significant hematological problems, the researchers noted. Studies have shown that lead interferes with heme biosynthesis, increases red cell destruction, and reduces gastrointestinal iron absorption, and lead toxicity has been linked with lower hemoglobin levels."

Let's pause for a definition some may need at this point. Hypocalcemia is too little calcium in the blood as determined by a blood test. In addition to keeping your bones and teeth strong, calcium is important to help your heart and muscles function properly. It also plays a role in the clotting of your blood and your nerve function.

None of this sounds particularly good. So, what do you do if you live in an area with 'acceptable' levels of lead in your water? The CDC suggests the following:

- "You can reduce or eliminate your exposure to lead in tap water by drinking or using only tap
- water that has been run through a "point-of-use" filter to reduce or eliminate lead (NSF/ANSI standard 53 for lead removal and NSF/ANSI standard 42 for particulate removal). If you have a lead service line, use a filter for all water you use for drinking or cooking.
- You can flush your water to reduce potential exposure to lead from household lead plumbing. This is especially important when the water has been off and sitting in the pipes for more than 6 hours. Before drinking, flush your home's pipes by running the tap, taking a shower, doing laundry, or doing a load of dishes. Drink or cook only with water that comes out of the tap cold. Water that comes out of the tap warm or hot can have higher levels of lead. Boiling this water will not reduce the amount of lead in your water.

- You can virtually eliminate your exposure to lead in water by drinking or using only bottled water that has been certified by an independent testing organization. This may not be the most cost-effective option for long-term use."

I'd had no idea how lead in the water affects advanced CKD patients. Did you?

5/30 *One Thing is Not Like the Other*

Here in the United States, today is Memorial Day. I'd like to take a minute to honor those who have died defending our freedom and let you know how glad I am that a certain Lieutenant Colonel (Retired) is not one of them. He's my husband, Bear. Thank you to all the soldiers of every race, religion, and sex who have kept us safe and died in the effort.

I explained the origins of this day in **SlowItDownCKD 2015** (May 25), so won't re-explain it here. You can go to the blog and just scroll down to that month and year in the drop-down menu on the right side of the page under Archives. I was surprised to read about the origins myself.

Now, let's look at not dying. Diabetes is the number one cause of chronic kidney disease. While this is not news to those of us with CKD or diabetes, I do have some information that is new to me. But let's start at the beginning. Do you remember the definition of diabetes? No? No problem. According to the CDC:

"Diabetes is a chronic (long-lasting) health condition that affects how your body turns food into energy.

Most of the food you eat is broken down into sugar (also called glucose) and released into your bloodstream. When your blood sugar goes up, it signals your pancreas to release insulin. Insulin acts like a key to let the blood sugar into your body's cells for use as energy.

If you have diabetes, your body either doesn't make enough insulin or can't use the insulin it makes as well as it should. When there isn't enough insulin or cells stop responding to insulin, too much blood sugar stays in your bloodstream. Over time, that can cause serious health problems, such as heart disease, vision loss, and kidney disease."

The American Diabetes Association tells us that appropriate levels of blood glucose for diabetics is an A1c [a blood test showing the average of your blood glucose over the previous three months] of over 7 is diabetic. Another way of testing is a finger prick of 70-130 before meals or above 180 after meals. It's this method of testing I want to write about today.

Okay, so what is this 'finger prick'? You actually make a hole in your finger to obtain a drop of blood. This hemoglobin is then tested via a blood test strip and a monitor. Here, VeryWellHealth will show you how it's done:

"Turn on the glucometer. This is usually done by inserting a test strip. The glucometer screen will tell you when it's time to put blood on the strip.

Use the lancing device to pierce the side of your finger, next to the fingernail (or another recommended location). This hurts less than lancing the pads of your fingers.

Squeeze your finger until it has produced a sufficent-size [sic] drop.

Place the drop of blood on the strip.

Blot your finger with the alcohol prep pad to stop the bleeding.

Wait a few moments for the glucometer to generate a reading."

The glucometer is the device. The test strip is what you apply your blood to. The lancet or lancing device is what pierces your skin. You can usually regulate the level of the needle on the lancet to find one that is less painful.

One thing I'd like you to remember is that this method tests hemoglobin.

I've previously explained that after losing two thirds of my pancreas to cancer, I was referred to the endocrinologist [specialist who deals with hormones of the body. Insulin is a hormone.] who suggested I might do better with insulin than I was doing with the oral medication. She also asked permission to prescribe a continuous monitoring device [CGM]. Wait. What was this?

WebMD explains:

"CGM measures the amount of glucose in the fluid inside your body. Different devices collect the information in different manners using tiny sensors. In some cases, the sensor is placed under the skin of your belly in a quick and painless fashion or, it can be adhered to the back of your arm. A transmitter on the sensor then sends the information to a wireless-pager-like monitor that you can clip on your belt.

The monitor displays your sugar levels at 1-, 5-, 10-, or 15-minute intervals. If your sugar drops to a dangerously low level or a high preset level, the monitor will sound an alarm."

Now, remember the glucometer tests your hemoglobin for blood glucose? The fluid mentioned in discussing the CGM is not your hemoglobin, but your blood serum. That was news to me and, for some reason, I found it fascinating. Now I understand how that little, teeny needle applied to my skin – I wear the CGM on the back of my arm – can read my blood glucose. It is also a tremendous relief to feel that prick once every two weeks, instead of several times a day. Well, sometimes I do have to use the glucometer and prick my finger to make certain the CGM is calibrated.

A few weeks ago, I promised to let you know when Cancer Dancer was published. Not only was it published last week, but Amazon deemed it the # 1 New Release in Chemotherapy. It garnered its first review that same week AND it was a five-star review!

6/6 *How Sweet We Need It*

I had an odd experience just the other day. While Bear was having a procedure on his poor back, I was in the waiting room. You know how it is; after a while, people start to talk to each other... even though we were six feet apart and masked. The woman across from me mentioned to her granddaughter that her blood sugar was crashing. I overheard and offered her some glucose tablets that I always carry with me in case my own blood glucose crashes. She was glad I offered but told me she used Advocate Glucose SOS. She saw the perplexed look on my face and handed over a packet for me to try.

That got me to thinking. Maybe there were other products for low blood sugar [Notice I'm using glucose and sugar interchangeably.] that I knew nothing about. Time to explore.

First let me remind you that diabetes is the foremost cause of chronic kidney disease. That's why I write about it sometimes... like today. Then I'd like to tell you about what I was using. Years ago, when I was pre-diabetic, a diabetes educator recommended CVS Health Glucose Tablets which were only $1.99 for 10 tablets. That worked for me since CVS was our local pharmacy, so I never explored anything else. They came in several flavors. I remember strawberry and orange. They were gluten, sodium, and fat free, although there was not only natural but also artificial flavoring. There were only four grams of carbohydrate and, of course, it was fast acting. Such products are only used if you can't get to food that will raise your blood sugar.

I know, I know. You're asking yourself what's the big deal about low blood glucose. The NIDDK defines it for us:

" Low blood glucose, also called low blood sugar or hypoglycemia [Gail here: another synonym], occurs when the level of glucose in your blood drops below what is healthy for you. For many people with diabetes, this means a blood glucose reading lower than 70 milligrams per deciliter (mg/dL) …. Your number might be different, so check with your doctor or health care team to find out what blood glucose level is low for you."

So? Why is this a big deal for diabetics? Healthline explains:

"Insufficient blood sugar levels can cause a rapid heartbeat and heart palpitations. However, even if you have diabetes, you may not always have obvious symptoms of low blood sugar. This is a potentially dangerous condition called hypoglycemia unawareness. It happens when you experience low blood sugar so often that it changes your body's response to it.

Normally, low blood sugar causes your body to release stress hormones, such as epinephrine. Epinephrine is responsible for those early warning signs, like hunger and shakiness.

When low blood sugar happens too frequently, your body may stop releasing stress hormones, called hypoglycemia-associated autonomic failure, or HAAF. That's why it's so important to check your blood sugar levels often."

This is more serious than I realized. Let's take a look at the product the lady in the waiting room used. All I got from their website is that it comes in four favors: green apple crisp, original sweet & tangy, fruit medley, and Kiwi-strawberry, and that it costs $10.99 for 6 packets. The packet itself gave me more information. What I liked is that there are "No artificial ingredients, colors, or flavors. Sodium and preservation free, caffeine and gluten free." It has 15 grams of carbohydrate per serving, which is what is usually recommended to raise your blood glucose. Nuts! It contains tricalcium phosphate, a form of phosphorous. Some of us with CKD need to limit our phosphorous.

I want to make it clear I am not endorsing these products, just letting you know of their existence. After all, I've only tried the CVS product.

WebMD tells us what to do if you have low blood sugar:

"First, eat or drink 15 grams of a fast-acting carbohydrate, such as:

- Three to four glucose tablets
- One tube of glucose gel
- Four to six pieces of hard candy (not sugar-free)
- 1/2 cup fruit juice
- 1 cup skim milk
- 1/2 cup soft drink (not sugar-free)
- 1 tablespoon honey (put it under your tongue so it gets absorbed into your bloodstream faster)

Fifteen minutes after you've eaten a food with sugar in it, check your blood sugar again. If your blood sugar is still less than 70 mg/dL, eat another serving of one of the foods listed above. Repeat these steps until your sugar becomes normal."

Aha! They recommend the products we're learning about today as well as certain foods. My diabetes/CKD nutritionist likes orange juice to raise my blood glucose but realizes I cannot always get it if I'm not home. That's why I carry a product with me at all times. I cringe at thinking of what might happen if I didn't have it in the car or my purse and had low blood glucose while I was driving.

Let's look at one more product. Amazon has Rite Aid glucose gummies in assorted fruit flavors. You get 60 pectin gummies for $7.28, but each is only two grams of carbohydrate. It might be fun. They remind me of candy. They're vegetarian, but aren't all blood glucose products? I really don't know, but it makes sense that they would be.

There are myriads of low blood sugar products available. While this was a surprise to me, it allows diabetics great choice.

Why shouldn't we ignore low blood glucose, I wondered. The American Diabetes Association had the answer… and it wasn't pretty.

"If the blood sugar glucose continues to drop, the brain does not get enough glucose and stops functioning as it should. This can lead to blurred vision, difficulty concentrating, confused thinking, slurred speech, numbness, and drowsiness. If blood glucose stays low for too long, starving the brain of glucose, it may lead to seizures, coma, and very rarely death."

Okay then. Those of us with diabetes, let's pay attention to our blood glucose levels.

6/13 *They Can be a Pair*

Last week, I was back in surgery... but for a welcome reason this time. After almost three years of remission, my oncologist felt it was safe to remove my PowerPort. That's where the harsh chemotherapy drugs entered my body. I was glad to have it gone because it was attached to my jugular vein and that made me nervous.

While I was in pre-op, one of the nurses looked at my chart and asked me about my chronic kidney disease. After I explained, she told me she had had a pancreas/kidney transplant. I was captivated to the point of almost being disappointed when it was time for my procedure, and she hadn't finished relating her story. So, I decided to do what I usually do. Research it myself.

I had all sorts of theories in my head about why the two might be transplanted together. I was curious to see if they were anywhere near the truth. The Mayo Clinic was helpful here:

"Combined kidney-pancreas transplant. Surgeons often may perform combined (simultaneous) kidney-pancreas transplants for people with diabetes who have or are at risk of kidney failure. Most pancreas transplants are done at the same time as a kidney transplant."

Aha! Not only does that make sense, but it was one of my theories. I have diabetes, type 2 and I have CKD. Does that make me a candidate for a pancreas/kidney transplant. Actually, since the pancreatic cancer, I only have the head of my pancreas, does that affect the situation?

I turned to The National Kidney Foundation to find out:

"Adults who have kidney failure because of type 1 diabetes are possible candidates for a kidney-pancreas transplant. In type 1 diabetes, the pancreas does not make enough insulin, a hormone that controls the blood sugar level in your body. The transplanted pancreas can make insulin and correct this type of diabetes.

In order to become active on the transplant waiting list you must be:

18 years or older

Have both Type 1 diabetes and kidney failure

Complete evaluation and be approved by transplant center for a kidney and pancreas transplant"

Well, that lets me out. Kidney failure is when your kidneys don't work well enough to keep you alive. My GFR has lowered since my cancer dance, but at 41%, the kidneys are still doing their job. Nor do I have type 1 diabetes, the kind in which your pancreas produces insufficient insulin. Although I only have the head of my pancreas remaining, I'm producing enough insulin to be insulin resistant. [Gee, how lucky for me, she thought sarcastically.]

The nurse I spoke with said her pancreas/kidney transplant had been redone. It was originally done the "old way" that caused her problems and needed to be done the "new way." That's when I was wheeled to the operating room. Darn! You know my curiosity was aroused. What was the old way? The new way? What problems had been caused by doing the operation the old way?

I came across this discussion in Pub Med Central's Annals of Surgery, May 1999:

"Dr. John C. McDonald (Shreveport, Louisiana): This is a detailed report on the current outcome of simultaneous kidney-pancreas transplantation, and is another fine presentation from the Memphis group… (which) has led the field in reestablishing the concept that best results are obtained when endocrine activity is delivered through the portal system and exocrine function through the GI tract. This concept was thought correct intuitively in the early efforts of transplanting the pancreas but was soon abandoned because of technical complications."

I needed a little assistance understanding it. I offer you the same assistance.

Endocrine means "relating to or denoting glands which secrete hormones or other products directly into the blood."

The portal system is "the system of blood vessels consisting of the portal vein with its tributaries and branches.

Exocrine? That's "relating to or denoting glands that secrete their products through ducts opening onto an epithelium rather than directly into the bloodstream."

Epithelium means "the thin tissue forming the outer layer of a body's surface and lining the alimentary canal and other hollow structures."

And, finally, the alimentary canal is "the whole passage along which food passes through the body from mouth to anus. It includes the esophagus, stomach, and intestines — that runs from the mouth to the anus."

I'd like to think I knew all this, but instead I need to thank the various dictionaries I consulted for these definitions. Now, the way I'm reading this discussion seems to be saying that the original method of delivering the blood containing the glandular production via the portal and the other glands' secretions via the GI tract. Hmmm, so first that was the best way to transplant the pancreas, then it wasn't, then it was again. Well, what came in between? Or, since this discussion is from 1999, is there a new method now?

This is from a MedlLinePlus article published last year:

"The person's diseased pancreas is not removed during the operation. The donor pancreas is usually placed in the right lower part of the person's abdomen. Blood vessels from the new pancreas are attached to the person's blood vessels. The donor duodenum (first part of the small intestine right after the stomach) is attached to the person's intestine or bladder."

Look at that. Blood to the blood and exocrine secretions to the epithelium. I think that's what the above means, but I wouldn't swear to it. Wait a minute. The nurse did say that the new pancreas had been attached to her intestine which caused her trouble. Then it was removed from the intestine to be reattached to the bladder, which rectified the situation for her. So, I guess the current method is the original.

I hate to leave you hanging, but I feel I just don't understand enough to explain any more. Hopefully, what I have written will be of some help to those facing, or curious about, a pancreas/kidney transplant. Although, I didn't really write much about a kidney transplant since I've written about that several times already.

6/20 *It's Just Not Fair*

We all know I'm a medical mess. But now, I'm a disgruntled medical mess. You see, when you take insulin, you gain weight. I have diabetes and I take insulin, so I gained weight. Healthline explains:

"Weight gain is a normal side effect of taking insulin. Insulin helps you manage your body sugar by assisting your cells in absorbing glucose (sugar). Without insulin, the cells of your body are unable to use sugar for energy. You'll eliminate the extra glucose in your bloodstream through your urine or have it stay in the blood, causing high blood sugar levels.

You may experience weight loss before you start insulin therapy. The loss of sugar in your urine takes water with it, so some of this weight loss is due to water loss.

Also, unmanaged diabetes can make you extra hungry. This can lead to eating an increased amount of food even when you start insulin therapy. And when you start insulin therapy and begin getting your blood sugar under control, the glucose in your body is absorbed and stored. This causes weight gain if the amount you eat is more than you need for the day."

Okay, I was warned by my endocrinologist. I didn't like it, but I wasn't going to waste the life that had just been saved for me. Pancreatic cancer, remember?

So, what is not fair? It seems there's a new drug you can take to lose weight when you're on insulin and are type 2 diabetes. Yay! I can't take it. Boo! I went to The Mayo Clinic to explore this drug and discovered more than I'd expected to:

"Some diabetes medications that help regulate blood glucose levels — including metformin (Fortamet, Glucophage, others), exenatide (Byetta), liraglutide (Victoza), albiglutide (Tarzeum), dulaglutide (Trulicity), sitagliptin (Januvia), saxagliptin (Onglyza), canagliflozin (Invokana), dapagliflozin (Farxiga), empagliflozin (Jardiance) and pramlintide (Symlin) — may promote weight loss and enable you to reduce your insulin dosage."

I was surprised that all of these might help with weight loss, but then I remembered I had tried several of them as a pre-diabetic and did not do well on them. It was a while ago, but nausea as a side effect sticks out in my mind.

I decided to do a search for the latest drug that both treated type 2 diabetes and helped with weight loss. Reminder: Type 1 diabetes is when you don't produce enough insulin and type 2 is when you are insulin resistant. Healthline provided this information:

"A once-weekly injectable recently approved to treat type 2 diabetes may hold major potential as a weight loss medication for people with obesity, too, a study suggests.

Overweight or obese participants without type 2 diabetes who took the drug, called tirzepatide (sold as the diabetes drug Mounjaro), lost an average of nearly 21 percent of their body weight at the highest dose studied. Scientists presented their findings at the American Diabetes Association (ADA)'s annual meeting in New Orleans and published the study in The New England Journal of Medicine.

'Definitely, the weight loss in this study is far more what we had ever seen with other FDA-approved medications in term of the absolute amount of weight lost or percentage of weight lost,' says Osama Hamdy, MD, PhD, an associate professor at Harvard Medical School and medical director of the obesity clinical program at the Joslin Diabetes Center in Boston....

Tirzepatide is the first drug in a new family of medicines that target two hormones — glucagon-like peptide-1 (GLP-1) and glucose-dependent insulinotropic polypeptide (GIP) — that are involved in maintaining healthy blood sugar levels and sending signals from the gut to the brain when people are full.

The U.S. Food and Drug Administration (FDA) approved tirzepatide in May to help manage blood sugar in people with type 2 diabetes; the diabetes treatment is called Mounjaro.

A head-to-head clinical trial found tirzepatide in this setting to be more effective at controlling blood sugar and spurring weight loss in type 2 diabetes patients than semaglutide (Ozempic), an injected GLP-1 receptor agonist, or two commonly used forms of insulin, according to the FDA.

In this earlier trial, tirzepatide reduced so-called hemoglobin A1C levels, which reflect average blood sugar levels over about three months, by 0.5 percent more than semaglutide and by about 1 percent more than insulin, the FDA said.

The 15 mg dose of tirzepatide helped type 2 diabetes patients with obesity lose 12 pounds more than semaglutide, and 27 to 29 pounds more than the two forms of insulin evaluated, the FDA noted."

I'm impressed, so much so that I wanted to try this new drug. My endocrinologist said no. I was disgruntled about that. She explained that I only have one quarter of my pancreas [and here I thought I had two thirds, but I hadn't realized the pancreas also has a neck. That was removed along with the body and tail leaving me only the head during the surgery to rid me of cancer.] So? What does that have to do with anything?

PharmarcyTimes supplied the answer:

"The drug has not been studied in patients with a history of pancreatitis and is not indicated for use in patients with type 1 diabetes mellitus, according to Eli Lilly."

Oh, I see. She wasn't willing to take the chance of damaging the remaining one quarter of my pancreas. I had never had pancreatitis but did have pancreatic cancer. This sounds like a case of don't poke the sleeping bear. I'll admit that I am leery of anything that may have the slightest chance of causing another cancer in my body.

6/27 *Dialysis & Transplant Change Your Renal Diet – Part 1*

I've spent so much time dwelling on how to combine the renal/diabetes diet that I've overlooked other big dietary changes for those of us who have chronic kidney disease. Several of my fellow CKD awareness advocates have had transplants. Some others are on dialysis. I am stage 3B. We all need to follow a renal diet, but they are not the same ones. I'm a little cautious about sharing the different diets since I know so little about them, but somebody's got to start somewhere with the differences. It might as well be me.

I'll start with the electrolytes I know about from my diet. Potassium is something I need to limit to about 2,000 mg. daily. According to the Collins Dictionary of Medicine, potassium is:

"An important body mineral present in carefully controlled concentration. Potassium is necessary for normal heart rhythm, for the regulation of the body's water balance and for the conduction of nerve impulses and the contraction of muscles."

If you're on dialysis, it's recommended you eat no more than 2,500 mg. daily, although some people may go as high as 3,000 mg. daily. Each person is different, so your nephrologist may urge you to keep your daily potassium at a different number.

And as a transplantee? The goal is 2,000 mg. daily, just as it is for pre-transplant CKD patients. Potassium can be problematic for those with a kidney transplant. Some of the immunosuppressive medications taken to prevent rejection of the new organ can raise their potassium level.

For the first time ever in my 14 years as a chronic kidney disease patient I have hyperkalemia or high potassium. That means I've got to avoid foods high in potassium such as those on WebMD's list:

"Many fresh fruits and vegetables are rich in potassium:

Bananas, oranges, cantaloupe, honeydew, apricots, grapefruit (some dried fruits, such as prunes, raisins, and dates, are also high in potassium)

Cooked spinach

Cooked broccoli

Potatoes

Sweet potatoes

Mushrooms

Peas

Cucumbers

Zucchini

Pumpkins

Leafy greens....

Orange juice

Tomato juice

Prune juice

Apricot juice

Grapefruit juice

Certain dairy products, such as milk and yogurt, are high in potassium (low-fat or fat-free is best).

Some fish contain potassium:

Tuna

Halibut

Cod

Trout

Rockfish

Beans or legumes that are high in potassium include:

Lima beans

Pinto beans

Kidney beans

Soybeans

Lentils

Other foods that are rich in potassium include:

Salt substitutes (read labels to check potassium levels)

Molasses

Nuts

Meat and poultry

Brown and wild rice

Bran cereal

Whole-wheat bread and pasta" There are exactly 16 items on this entire list that I don't eat. It's almost as if I have a potassium-based diet! Okay, changes coming… and quickly. That potassium is now listed on food labels will be helpful.

In my first CKD book, **What Is It and How Did I Get it? Early Stage Chronic Kidney Disease**, I called the dietary restrictions "the three p's and one s." Let's move on to another p, phosphorous. I am restricted to 800 mg. daily. According to verywellhealth:

"Phosphorus is an essential mineral found in every cell of the human body. It is the second most abundant mineral next to calcium, accounting for about 1% of your total body weight. Phosphorus is one of 16 essential minerals that your body needs to function properly.

Although the main purpose of phosphorus is to build and maintain bones and teeth, it also plays a major role in the formation of DNA and RNA (the genetic building blocks of the body). Doing so helps ensure that cells and tissues are properly maintained, repaired, and replaced as they age.

Phosphorus also plays a key role in metabolism (the conversion of calories and oxygen to energy), muscle contraction, heart rhythm, and the transmission of nerve signals. Phosphorus is considered a macromineral (along with calcium, sodium, magnesium, potassium, chloride, and sulfur) in that you need more of it than trace minerals like iron and zinc."

I'm doing well at controlling my phosphorous via diet. I also look for these ingredients on food labels since phosphorous itself is not listed:

Phosphorus additives found in foods include:

Dicalcium phosphate.

Disodium phosphate.

Monosodium phosphate.

Phosphoric acid.

Sodium hexameta-phosphate.

Trisodium phosphate.

Sodium tripolyphosphate.

Tetrasodium pyrophosphate.

Thank you to the National Kidney Foundation for the above list.

Let's see how dialysis deals with phosphorous. DaVita tells us:

"Neither hemodialysis or peritoneal dilaysis [sic] (PD) are very effective at eliminating phosphorus from the body. The amount of phosphorus removed in a dialysis treatment ranges from 250 to 1,000 mg per treatment. This number is affected by the pre-dialysis phosphorus level, the type of dialyzer and the amount of dialysis received."

I could not find a specific goal number for phosphorous when you are on dialysis, but most of the sites I looked at mentioned that your doctor will be watching your phosphorus levels with weekly blood tests. This is also when binders may come into play. Where else to go for a good definition of binders than Drugs.com?

"Phosphate binders are used to decrease the absorption of phosphate from food in the digestive tract.

They are used when there is an abnormally high blood phosphate level (hyperphosphatemia) which can be caused by impaired renal phosphate excretion or increased extracellular fluid phosphate loads.

Phosphate binders react with phosphate to form an insoluble compound, making it unable to be absorbed from the gastrointestinal tract. When taken regularly with meals, phosphate binders lower the concentration of phosphate in serum."

Transplantees need to be careful since their immunosuppressant medications may raise their phosphorous levels. You'll have to watch your diet, too. Healthline tells us some high phosphorous foods that need to be either cut out of your diet or minimized in your diet are:

Dairy foods.

Beans.

Lentils.

Nuts.

Bran cereals.

Oatmeal.

Colas and other drinks with phosphate additives.

Some bottled ice tea.

It looks like this blog will have to be a two parter, or maybe a series. You can see I anticipated that in the title of this blog. Here I am offering the most basic information about dietary changes for CKD, dialysis, and transplant and there's an awful lot of that, basic or not.

7/4 *Dialysis & Transplant Change Your Renal Diet – Part 2*

Before we start, let's acknowledge that today is Independence Day in the U.S. For those not in the U.S., it's the day we celebrate Congress's Declaration of Independence from England back in 1776. The Second Continental Congress had ratified our independence just two days earlier. The most usual celebration is a fireworks display accompanied by a backyard bar-b-q with friends and family.

That's an easy transition to writing about your kidney [renal] diet no matter if you're a chronic kidney disease stages 1-5 patient, a dialysis patient, or a transplantee. Last week, I wrote about two of the three p's as I called them in my first CKD book *What Is It and How Did I Get It? Early Stage Chronic Kidney Disease.* Those are the electrolytes potassium and phosphorous.

Last week, I neglected to define electrolyte. MedlinePlus can rectify that right now:

"Electrolytes are minerals in your blood and other body fluids that carry an electric charge.

Electrolytes affect how your body functions in many ways, including:

The amount of water in your body

The acidity of your blood (pH)

Your muscle function

Other important processes

You lose electrolytes when you sweat. You must replace them by drinking fluids that contain electrolytes. Water does not contain electrolytes."

I can practically hear you asking what electrolytes have to do with your kidneys. I turned to verywellhealth for an explanation we can all understand:

"Electrolyte abnormalities are very common in kidney disease states for one simple reason—it is the kidney that typically has a central role in maintaining normal levels of most electrolytes. Therefore, these abnormalities are a consequence of abnormal kidney function, rather than a cause.

Both low and high levels of electrolytes can be seen when the kidneys malfunction...."

Aha! So, we've got to keep our kidneys as healthy as possible to control our electrolytes. It is a little too late to keep our electrolytes normal if we already have CKD, are on dialysis, or have a transplant. However, there's no reason not to try. I think I already mentioned at one point that I have hyperkalemia [high potassium] for the first time. I also have a significantly lower GFR than I'm used to. You see where I'm going with this?

Okay, let's get to that third 'p' I mentioned. It's protein. As stage 3B, I am restricted to five ounces a day. Since I've never had either high or low protein on my blood tests, I wonder if I am automatically sticking to that restriction. I honestly doubt it, so I'll have to do better. Protein is hard on the kidneys.

It's a good thing that the National Kidney Foundation explains why so well:

"Your body needs protein to help build muscle, repair tissue, and fight infection. If you have kidney disease, you may need to watch how much protein you eat. Having too much protein can cause waste to build up in your blood, and your kidneys may not be able to remove all the extra waste. If protein intake is too low, however, it may cause other problems so it is essential to eat the right amount each day.

The amount of protein you need is based on:

your body size

your kidney problem

the amount of protein in your urine

Your dietitian or healthcare provider can tell you how much protein you should eat."

Luckily for me, I'll be seeing my nephrologist later this week and will be sure to ask him how much protein I should be having on a daily basis. Due to the diabetes, I have gained weight. Perhaps that changed the amount of protein I should be having daily. We'll see. Then again, there's that change in my GFR. What will that change? Of course, I won't know the amount of protein in my urine until I see the results from the blood tests I took previous to this appointment.

I like to know exactly what happens in my kidneys, so let's see what too little or too much protein can do to them. The Journal of the American Society of Nephrology has an explanation that is surprisingly easy for laypeople [that's us: non-doctors] to understand:

"Although there has not been a full elucidation of the underlying mechanisms by which high protein intake may adversely affect kidney function, particularly in the context of CKD, existing data suggest that glomerular hyperfiltration caused by a high-protein diet may lead to an increase in albuminuria and an initial rise and subsequent decline in GFR …. Furthermore, growing evidence suggests that high-protein diets may be associated with a number of metabolic complications that may be detrimental to kidney health."

Reminder: albuminuria and proteinuria are not the same thing.

Let's take a look at the protein needs for dialysis patients. I found this on DaVita's website:

"Excess protein waste can cause nausea, loss of appetite, vomiting, weakness, taste changes and itching.... Dialysis removes protein waste from the blood and a low protein diet is no longer needed.

Unfortunately, some amino acids are removed during dialysis. A higher protein intake is needed to replace lost protein."

What about protein needs after a transplant? The University of Michigan was more than helpful here:

"For the first 6-8 weeks after transplant, you will need a high protein diet to help heal. Dialysis patients will need as much or more protein following transplant than they did during dialysis. Chronic Kidney Disease (CKD) patients not on dialysis will definitely require more protein after transplant. Protein is important for healing and strength. High doses of prednisone can cause muscle breakdown, making adequate protein intake even more crucial. Six to 8 weeks after the transplant, you should reduce protein intake to 6 to 8 ounces daily."

I thought we needed a little humor here, so I've included Australia's Betterhealth list of protein foods:

"lean meats – beef, lamb, veal, pork, kangaroo

poultry – chicken, turkey, duck, emu, goose, bush birds

fish and seafood – fish, prawns, crab, lobster, mussels, oysters, scallops, clams

eggs

dairy products – milk, yoghurt (especially Greek yoghurt), cheese (especially cottage cheese)

nuts (including nut pastes) and seeds – almonds, pine nuts, walnuts, macadamias, hazelnuts, cashews, pumpkin seeds, sesame seeds, sunflower seeds

legumes and beans – all beans, lentils, chickpeas, split peas, tofu."

There's so much difference in the dietary needs amongst CKD, dialysis, and transplant patients… and we haven't even dealt with the 's' in the '3 p's and 1 s.' That's sodium or, as we usually refer to it, salt although there is a difference between the two. That will be part 3 in this series.

7/11 *Dialysis & Transplant Change Your Renal Diet – Part 3*

Here's hoping you had a nice, quiet, safe July 4th, Canada Day, or whatever holiday your country celebrates. Here's hoping you were able to adhere to your renal diet, too. As I told one reader years ago when she was overwhelmed by the dietary changes she had to make, make one change at a time if you have to. You'll get there.

Let's see now. This topic has definitely turned into a series instead of a two parter. In the last two blogs, I wrote about the three 'p's as I called them in my first CKD book, What Is It and How Did I Get It? Early Stage Chronic Kidney Disease. These are phosphorous, potassium, and protein. Guess that leaves the one 's' in the renal diet. I made mention last week that sodium and salt are not exactly the same thing, so let's look at that first.

Thank you to WebMd for this explanation:

"Sodium is a type of metal that is always found as a salt. The most common dietary form is sodium chloride. Sodium chloride is commonly called table salt.

Table salt accounts for 90% of dietary sodium intake in the US. Sodium helps to balance levels of fluids and electrolytes in the body. This balance can affect blood pressure and the health of the kidneys and heart."

A usual restriction for CKD patients is 2000 mg./day. That's where I am, too. Although, I have seen 2,300 mg./day for men.

Hmmm, how does sodium "affect blood pressure and the health of the kidneys and heart." The more I blog, the more I want to know the how. I turned to The American Stroke Association:

"'With the circulatory system, salt's effects are a very simple plumbing problem,' said Dr. Fernando Elijovich, a professor of medicine at Vanderbilt University.

The heart is the pump and blood vessels are the pipes, he said. Blood pressure goes up if you increase how much blood has to move through the pipes. Blood pressure also rises if you shrink those pipes.

Salt does both. When there's excess salt in your system, the heart pumps more blood in a given time, boosting blood pressure. And over time, salt narrows the vessels themselves, which is the most common 'plumbing' feature of high blood pressure.

The harm can come quickly. And over time.

Within 30 minutes of eating excess salt, your blood vessels' ability to dilate is impaired, Elijovich said. The damage from persistent high blood pressure shows up down the road, in the form of heart attacks, strokes and other problems.

The good news, Laffer said, is the benefits of cutting back on excess salt also show up quickly. If you significantly reduce how much salt you eat, your blood pressure goes down within hours or days."

Do you remember that high blood pressure is one of the leading causes of CKD? With CKD, your kidneys do not function well and filter out less sodium. This seems circular. You develop high blood pressure from too much sodium and then develop chronic kidney disease. Your kidneys no longer effectively function so you excrete less sodium… which raises your blood pressure even more.

This much I know because I'm stage 3A CKD. I was 3B when I wrote the first two parts of this series. I believe increased hydration brought me up to 3A again, but that has nothing to do with sodium. Or does it?

And in dialysis? DaVita Kidney Care has this to say about sodium restriction in dialysis:

"If you have stage 5 CKD and require dialysis, you will be asked to follow a low-sodium diet. The diet will help control blood pressure and fluid intake. Controlling sodium intake will help avoid cramping and blood pressure drops during dialysis. Your dietitian will determine how much sodium you can eat each day and counsel you on regulating it in your diet."

Finally, let's look at sodium restrictions for transplantees. I automatically went to the National Kidney Foundation:

"Most people still need to limit salt after they get a transplant, although it is different with each person. Transplant medicines, especially steroids, may cause your body to hold on to fluid, and salt makes this problem worse. Increased fluid in the body raises blood pressure. Controlling blood pressure is very important to your transplant. Your doctor will decide how much sodium is best for you. It is a good idea to limit foods high in salt, such as:

Table salt

Cured meats, such as ham, bacon, and sausage

Lunch meats, such as bologna, salami, and hot dogs

Pre-packaged frozen dinners

Ramen noodles, boxed noodles, and potato and rice mixes

Canned soups and pasta sauce

Pickled foods, such as olives, pickles, and sauerkraut

Snack foods, such as salted chips, nuts, pretzels, and popcorn"

I love learning as I write these blogs. The thing that surprised me most was why dialysis patients need to restrict their sodium intake. I think I need to learn more about dialysis.

7/18 *Did You Say Portable?*

Way back in February of last year, I wrote about the Phase 1 KidneyX competition. Now we have the Phase 1 winner. Oh, you've forgotten what KidneyX is? No problem. This is from the previously mentioned blog:

"The Kidney Innovation Accelerator (KidneyX), a public-private partnership between the U.S. Department of Health and Human Services (HHS) and the American Society of Nephrology (ASN), is accelerating innovation in the prevention, diagnosis, and treatment of kidney diseases."

According to USA.gov, "The U.S. Department of Health and Human Services protects the health of all Americans and provides essential human services." The American Society of Nephrology (ASN) is self-explanatory. The two working together present a powerful front.

This was posted on the KidneyX Prize Winner's site:

"Winner: Development Of A Dialysate-Free Waterless Portable And Implantable Artificial Kidney

Winning Submission

We have created a portable artificial kidney device that fits into a backpack that can be used at night or at work while sitting on a nearby table. Moreover, taking advantage of the fact that the device does not need water or dialysate, we will use the same technology to create for the first time a completely implantable artificial kidney. Patients are very enthusiastic about our portable and implantable artificial kidney devices because they offer more personalized treatment than dialysis and because of the more accurate ability to control fluctuations in toxins to be removed. Importantly patients are also excited about the improvement in their quality of life because of the ability to use the device at home or at work coupled with the increased ease of treatment. In addition, for patients who chose to remain on peritoneal dialysis, our technology offers the advantage of decreasing the number of treatment fluid exchanges needed. The important advantages of our technology to patients include: 1) Since the use of the device occurs at night or during the day at home or at work, patients will no longer need to go to a dialysis clinic and will have increased mobility to travel and work; 2) The technology will provide patients with more treatment options; 2) Dialysate solutions, large R/O water tanks and large storage space for home modalities will no longer be needed decreasing the overall cost of treatment; 3) Given the potential for greater clearances and efficiency of treatment, the diet and fluid intake can be liberalized; 4) In its ultimately implantable format, patients will be entirely mobile and not require a CVC line or access; 5) Given the shortage of kidneys for transplant, patients who have dreamt for years of getting off dialysis will now be offered this opportunity.

Submitter Bio

Ira Kurtz, MD, FRCP, FASN, is Distinguished Professor of Medicine, Chief of the Division of Nephrology, Factor Chair, and a member of the University of California, Los Angeles (UCLA) Brain Research Institute. Dr. Kurtz is a scientific and medical advisor for US Kidney Research Corporation for the development of a portable and implantable artificial kidney. Dr. Kurtz is a graduate of the University of Toronto and completed his postgraduate training at both the University of California, San Francisco, and the National Institutes of Health. Dr. Kurtz has been a faculty member at UCLA since 1985 and is board-certified in Internal Medicine by the American Board of Internal Medicine and in Nephrology by the American Board of Nephrology. Dr. Kurtz is a Fellow of the Royal College of Physicians and Surgeons of Canada, and the American Society of

Nephrology, and is listed in Southern California Super Doctors. He is a member of the American Society of Clinical Investigation, the American Physiological Society, the Biophysical Society, and the American Society of Nephrology. Dr. Kurtz has authored over 300 scientific publications, book chapters, and abstracts. He is on the editorial board of several scientific journals and is an external reviewer of major scientific publications and grants. Dr. Kurtz's primary areas of research include ion transport-related diseases, the physiology and biophysics of molecular transport processes in the kidney and extrarenal organs, structural biology, the atomic structure of membrane proteins, and the development of an artificial kidney.

Since I am not on dialysis, I needed some terms explained. Maybe you do, too.

CVC line: A central venous catheter is a thin, flexible tube that is inserted into a vein, usually below the right collarbone, and guided (threaded) into a large vein above the right side of the heart called the superior vena cava. It is used to give intravenous fluids, blood transfusions, chemotherapy, and other drugs. [This definition is from the National Cancer Institute. Those following are from Merriam-Webster Dictionary.]

Dialysate: the material that passes through the membrane in dialysis

peritoneum: the smooth transparent serous membrane that lines the cavity of the abdomen of a mammal and is folded inward over the abdominal and pelvic viscera

peritoneal dialysis: a procedure performed in the peritoneal cavity in which the peritoneum acts as the semipermeable membrane

Putting myself in what I think might be the mindset of a dialysis patient, I am filled with hope at the thought of possibly making my life easier and allowing me to work again. I'd like to hear from actual dialysis patients to get your take on this new machine.'

But wait; there's more. In Tina Daunt's interview on UCLA Health, Dr. Kurtz tells us:

"'The device we're working on is complicated,' Dr. Kurtz said. 'We have four separate components in it. The first component is called the ultrafiltration module, and it filters the blood. By filtering the blood, what I mean is that it prevents the cells in the blood and proteins from getting into the rest of the device'....

There are additional components in the device, including a nanofiltration module to prevent the excretion of sugar in the artificial urine and two custom-designed electrodeionization modules that transport various ions into the synthetic urine. One of the electrodeionization modules is specific for potassium.

'If your blood potassium changes by just a little bit, the electricity in your heart can just go wacko and your heart can stop,' Dr. Kurtz said. 'So it's very important that we keep the potassium in the blood within a certain range.'

Finally, the device includes a reverse osmosis module that ensures the appropriate amount of water is excreted in the synthetic urine....

Dr. Kurtz estimates that his team needs another 18 months to refine the technology on the wearable artificial kidney and then will focus on the implantable artificial kidney...."

18 months. The article was printed in January of last year. We are soooo close.

7/25 *Nailed It!*

Every so often, my friend Geo often asks pertinent questions or tells me about something he's read. This week he told me about an article he'd read on nail fungus and CKD. My initial reaction was to wonder what nail fungus could possibly have to do with chronic kidney disease. Of course, what followed was my determination to find out.

Let's start with nail fungus. I found the Mayo Clinic has a good explanation:

"Nail fungus is a common condition that begins as a white or yellow spot under the tip of your fingernail or toenail. As the fungal infection goes deeper, nail fungus may cause your nail to discolor, thicken and crumble at the edge. It can affect several nails.

If your condition is mild and not bothering you, you may not need treatment. If your nail fungus is painful and has caused thickened nails, self-care steps and medications may help. But even if treatment is successful, nail fungus often comes back.

Nail fungus is also called onychomycosis (on-ih-koh-my-KOH-sis). When fungus infects the areas between your toes and the skin of your feet, it's called athlete's foot (tinea pedis)."

I think we need one more thing before we see how CKD is involved and that is the definition of fungus. I was surprised to discover that the National Cancer Institute had the most easily understood definition of the term:

"A plant-like organism that does not make chlorophyll. Mushrooms, yeasts, and molds are examples. The plural is fungi."

The thought of something like that growing on my nails is more than a little creepy. What's even creepier is that CKD might have something to do with it.

I found this on ResearchGate:

"Abnormalities of the skin and its appendage are commonly encountered in renal patients.... Other frequently observed onychomycopathies in CKD patients include onychomycosis, onycholysis, leukonychia, clubbing, and brittle nails. Onychomycosis, a commonly encountered fungal infection, also often manifests among CKD patients. Nail diseases in patients on maintenance hemodialysis are common and may affect up to 71.4 % of these patients. There is no direct relation between the dose and duration of hemodialysis and the increased prevalence of nail abnormalities. A significant incidence of nail changes among renal transplant recipients has also been described with a reported overall frequency of 56.6 %. Nail pathology increases with age and correlates with longer duration of immunosuppression. The most commonly encountered nail changes in renal transplant recipients include leukonychia, absence of lunula, onychomycosis, longitudinal ridging, and Muehrcke lines."

Now before you start wondering why I'm taxing you with all these medical terms, the only one you need to deal with is "onychomycosis," which, as the Mayo Clinic has already explained, is also called nail fungus.

Seems pretty clear to me so far... except for what CKD has to do with it. The Global Nail Fungus Organization remedied that problem:

"CKD patients may experience abnormal fingernail and toenail changes due to malnutrition. Nails are made up of protein, which people suffering from chronic kidney disease are likely lacking of in their diet. As damaged kidneys lose their ability to excrete wastes and toxins out of the body, they cause sufferers to lose vitamins and other nutrition, all of which are necessary for healthy growth of nails. They are also at high risk of zinc deficiency, which is related to nail changes.

Therefore, CKD sufferers often experience abnormal nail changes, which include getting brittle nails, pitted nails, yellow or white coloring, and white streaks or spots on the nails. The most common nail disorders people with CKD often get are absent lunula (the crescent-shaped white area of the bed of a nail) and half and half nails (half white and half red, pink or brown color appearance of the nail with an apparent demarcation line).

Since abnormal changes to the nail are consequences of having chronic kidney disease, even with known nail treatments, the nails are unlikely to go back to normal unless the kidney disease is treated successfully.

Onychomycosis in Patients with Chronic Renal Failure

Patients with chronic renal failure may also experience onychomycosis, or nail fungi infection. In one study aiming to assess the frequency of onychomycosis in CKD patients undergoing hemodialysis (the process of filtering wastes and other toxins from the body using a machine), it found out that the frequency of nail fungi infection among the 100 patients was 39%. The risk of acquiring the onychomycosis went up by 1.9% for each additional year in age, with diabetic patients 88% more likely to develop the infection than non-diabetic patients.

The study did not find the association of the development of onychomycosis with the duration of hemodialysis treatment."

Conversely, our nails can tip us off that we have kidney disease. Walk-In Lab explains:

"When people have kidney disease, nitrogen waste products build up in our bodies. Your kidneys are not filtering those products out properly. This can lead to changes in the look and structure of both fingernails and toenails. It's not the ONLY cause of change though. Malnutrition and taking some medications can also contribute....

There are three different types of nails to be on the lookout for when it specifically comes to chronic kidney disease.

Beau's lines

The name comes from a French physician, Joseph Honore Simon Beau, who first described the condition in 1846. Beau's lines are deep grooved lines that run horizontally from side to side on the finger or toenail.... These can be signs of acute kidney disease that interferes with the growth of the nail. They can also be signs of diabetes and vascular disease.

Ridged nails

The official name for this is koilonychia. These are rough looking nails with ridges that are frequently spoon-shaped and concave. In the early stages of this condition, the nails may be brittle, chipping easily. Ridged nails happen when you have iron-deficiency anemia.... These type of nails can also be a sign of heart disease or hypothyroidism.

White streaks/spots

The medical name for this type of nail is leukonychia, which comes from the Greek words that mean 'white nails.' This is when white lines or dots appear on your finger or toenails. They can be many dots on one nail or it might be one larger spot that stretches across the nail.... Injury is the largest cause of white spots, but they can also be indicative of heart disease, psoriasis and arsenic poisoning, as well as kidney disease.

Other things to look for in nails are loosening nails, black lines, redness around the nail bed, half-and-half nails (also known as Lindsay's nails) as they can indicate other diseases besides kidney disease.
If you look down at your nails and see any of these patterns, check with your local healthcare provider. They may want to run tests on you to see if it's something minor or the start of something serious."

Well, I'm glad Geo asked. I suspected there was a connection but hadn't expected it to be so complex.

8/1 *They Go Together*

Let me tell you how today's topic came into being first. My cousin, Dan Bernard, has a podcast called Human BioSciences. He decided to interview me. I was onboard from day one. The interview was released last week. As I was listening to it, I heard myself tell the story of the nurse who noticed I had chronic kidney disease and started to tell me about her pancreas/kidney transplant. Oh, you can listen to the podcast, too, at https://humanbiosciences.com/woundcarepodcast. Anyway, she never got to finish her story because it was my turn for surgery.

I have CKD and I had ¾ of my pancreas removed due to cancer. I was stymied. Why both of these organs? What was the connection? Why [how?] did they go together? That's what I intend to discover today. We all know what the kidneys are… otherwise why read my blog? But what about the pancreas?

On June 13 of this year, I wrote about the pancreas/kidney transplant and how it's done. What I didn't write about was how the two organs work together. That's what we'll find out today.

Just in case you're not sure what the pancreas is, MedicineNet will help us out:

"The pancreas, which is about the size of a hand, is located in the abdomen, just behind the stomach. It is surrounded by other organs including the small Intestine, liver, and spleen. [Lost my spleen, also, during the cancer surgery.] The pancreas plays a vital role in converting the food into energy. It mainly performs two functions: an exocrine function [That means the secretion it produces is released outside its source.] that helps in digestion and an endocrine function [This means the hormone is released directly into the blood stream.] that controls blood sugar levels.

Because of the deep location of the pancreas, tumors of the pancreas may be difficult to locate.

The exocrine pancreas produces natural juices called pancreatic enzymes to break down food. These enzymes travel through the tubes or ducts to reach the duodenum. [That's the part of the small intestine located below the stomach.] The pancreas makes about eight ounces of digestive juices filled with enzymes every day. The different enzymes are as follows:

Lipase: Along with bile, these enzymes break down fats. Poor absorption of fats leads to diarrhea and fatty bowel movements.

Protease: It breaks down proteins and builds immunity against the bacteria and yeast present in the intestine. Poor absorption of proteins can cause allergies.

Amylase: It helps to break down starch into sugar, which is then converted to energy to meet the body's demand. Undigested carbohydrates can cause diarrhea.

Unlike enzymes, hormones are released directly into the bloodstream. Pancreatic hormones include:

Insulin: This hormone is produced in the beta cells of the pancreas and helps the body to use sugar as the energy source. Lack of insulin can increase blood sugar levels in the blood and cause serious diseases such as diabetes.

Glucagon: Alpha cells produce the hormone glucagon. If blood sugar gets too low, glucagon helps to increase it by sending a message to the liver to release the stored sugar.

Amylin: A hormone called amylin is made in the beta cells of the pancreas. This helps in controlling our appetite (eating behavior)."

That's a pretty thorough explanation of the pancreas. Now let's see if we can figure out the connection between the pancreas and the kidneys.

MedlinePlus succinctly provided the answer:

"Uncontrolled diabetes causes damage to many tissues of the body including the kidneys. Kidney damage caused by diabetes most often involves thickening and hardening of the internal kidney structures. Strict blood glucose control may delay the progression of kidney disease in type 1 and type 2 diabetics."

Aha! Diabetes is caused by resistance to the insulin produced by the pancreas or the pancreas not producing insulin. If the insides of your kidneys harden or thicken, you're simply not getting your blood as clean as it could be.

Whoa! While I've been paying attention to controlling my blood sugar, I have to admit it hasn't been strict control. You know, it's a special occasion or I think "just once," and so indulge in carbs. Guess I'll have to stop that now that I know better. You, too?

Talking about carbohydrates, my diabetes/kidney dietitian mentioned a new [to me] product: Magic Spoon. The cereal has zero sugar, 5 grams of net carbs and 13 of protein. It's both grain and gluten free. Unfortunately, I am not a fan. However, you might be. As best as I can figure out from their website, you can choose your own flavors for variety packs. Here's what the company has to say for itself:

"Hi, we're Greg and Gabi, co-founders of Magic Spoon.

We've been friends for ten years: met at college, lived together, even started a previous business together (you could call us 'cereal' entrepreneurs...). We both grew up eating cereal every morning for breakfast, binging on the sugary crunch of the classic brands and then crashing from the empty carbs in the afternoon when we were supposed to be at our most productive.

Now that we're adults, we've searched for years for a cereal that has the same addictive quality as those sugar/corn bombs but actually fuels us for a healthy day. We've turned up nothing.

Plus, as we learned more about the cereal industry, we were shocked by the true scope of the problem. The average American eats 100 bowls of cereal a year (this even includes people who don't eat a single bowl!), and kids are one of the largest consumers. Yet almost every version in the aisle is stuck in that old paradigm of grains, empty carbs, and sugar.

We experimented for over a year to create a cereal inspired by the flavors and nostalgia of Saturday-morning-cartoon cereal but upgraded for a 21st-century consumer. A guilt-free treat that tastes like you remember and you can eat at any time of day...."

8/8 *What's Your Superpower?*

Last week, I mentioned that my renal/diabetes dietician had suggested Magic Spoon cereal since it's low carbohydrate. I didn't care for it. Marc Hernandez of Uhling Consulting was surprised, since he and his family really liked it. We tried to figure out why I didn't. Then Marc hit on something. Maybe I was a super taster. Oh goody, a new concept for me.

Let's get a definition for super taster before we go any further. According to Healthline, a super taster is

"... a person who tastes certain flavors and foods more strongly than other people."

Well, that's obvious. We need more. And that's what I discovered on LiveScience:

"... The tally of little mushroom-shaped projections on the tongue, called fungiform papillae, reveals a person's tasting prowess or deficit.

Nestled within the walls of these tiny bumps are our taste receptors, called taste buds, which register the five currently recognized tastes: bitterness, saltiness, sourness, sweetness and umami (savoriness). Touch receptors in the fungiform papillae also help us 'feel' our food's texture and temperature.

The application of blue food coloring makes the papillae easier to count. In a 6-millimeter diameter circle, which is 'about the size of a hole punch,' Bartoshuk said, supertasters can have as many as 60 fungiform papillae packed into the small space; nontasters can have as few as five."

Wait, there's more information from the discoverer and coiner of the term super tasters from CBC Radio:

"In Bartoshuk's research, she found that 25 per cent of people are incredibly sensitive to a bitter tasting chemical known as 6-n-propylthiouracil, or PROP. Another 25 per cent, deemed non-tasters, can't detect PROP at all, she says, while the remaining 50 per cent are considered average tasters.

While affixing super to anything sounds great, being a supertaster can actually be quite difficult, says Bartoshuk, who coined the terms supertaster and non-taster.

Supertasters are differentially more sensitive to bitter. Having more tastebuds means there are also more pain receptors, and that's why supertasters often can't handle spicy foods and generally avoid anything bitter. As a result, they are often seen as picky eaters.

However, their aversion to bitterness is evolutionary, says Bartoshuk.

'Supertasters are differentially more sensitive to bitter' than the average person.

Bartoshuk says there are 25 different bitter genes expressing 25 different bitter receptors.

'Why would nature do that? Because bitter is our poison detection system.'"

So, do I feel honored or cursed to possibly be a super taster? I think I need more information.

Wow! While more testing is needed, I found this article on National Geographic encouraging:

"Henry Barham, a rhinologist at the Baton Rouge General Medical Center, in Louisiana, published a study in the medical journal JAMA Network Open on May 25 that analyzed nearly 2,000 patients and found that 'supertasters'—individuals who are overly sensitive to some bitter compounds—were less likely to test positive for the virus. If this association holds true, it implies, for example, that people who don't find broccoli too bitter are in a higher risk group for severe COVID-19.

'This is a very interesting study that suggests that receptors on our tongue that allow us to sense bitter flavors are also linked to our vulnerability to respiratory infections like COVID-19,' says David Aronoff, director of the division of infectious diseases at Vanderbilt University Medical Center, in Nashville, Tennessee, who was not involved with this research. That taste receptors may also be involved with immunity is surprising, he says….

According to Aronoff, the study has limitations. The relatively small number of adults examined were in a fairly narrow age range, so it's not known whether the correlation between taste preferences and COVID-19 severity exists in children or the elderly. In addition, he says, the population studied may differ in unknown ways that influenced the results."

Hmmm, and that has to do with the renal diet or diabetes how? Back to Healthline for the answer:

"Pros of being a supertaster:

May weigh less than average or non-tasters. That's because supertasters often avoid sugary, fatty foods that are often packed with calories. These flavors can be too overwhelming and unenjoyable, just like bitter flavors.

Are less likely to drink and smoke. The bittersweet flavors of beer and alcohol are often too bitter for supertasters. Plus, the flavor of smoke and tobacco can be too harsh, too.

Cons of being a supertaster

Eat few healthy vegetables. Cruciferous vegetables, including Brussels sprouts, broccoli, and cauliflower, are very healthy. Supertasters often avoid them, however, because of their bitter flavors. This can lead to vitamin deficiencies.

May be at a higher risk for colon cancer. The cruciferous vegetables they can't tolerate are important for digestive health and helping lower the risk of certain cancers. People who don't eat them may have more colon polyps and higher cancer risks.

May have an increased risk for heart disease. Salt masks bitter flavors, so supertasters tend to use it on many foods. Too much salt, however, can cause health problems, including high blood pressure and heart disease.

May be picky eaters. Foods that are too bitter just aren't pleasant. That limits the number of foods many supertasters will eat."

Here are some reminders to help you see the connections.

Pros:

Obesity can lead to diabetes. Smoking and drinking can hasten your CKD.

Cons:

SALT! The bane of CKD. Also, being picky means you may not be fulfilling your nutritional needs and, instead filling up on foods that will only worsen your CKD and/or diabetes.

After all this researching, I've come to the conclusion that I am not among the 25% of the population that are super tasters. Nor am I part of the 25% of non-tasters. Yep, I'm part of the 50% of average tasters. I just happen not to care for the taste of Magic Spoon. Again, that doesn't mean you won't. After all, Marc and his family like it.

8/15 Move It (Please)

Lately, everywhere I look I see some information about exercise. That's probably because I've had enough of hiding from it. I didn't feel like I had much control over my pancreatic cancer, but I did have control over whether I exercised or not. So, I didn't. Bad move on my part. It's taken me almost three years to understand that I wasn't doing myself any favors by avoiding exercise.

So first, I tried tap dancing. I'd always wanted to learn how to do that. Gregory Hines was my hero at one time just because he was such a marvelous tap dancer. That didn't work out too well. I have osteoarthritis in my feet, knees, and hips. My rheumatologist strongly suggested I NOT tap dance. Oh, well.

Then I thought I'd go back to walking. I used to love to take my dog on long, wandering walks. Unfortunately, Sweet Ms. Bella succumbed to her own cancer. A few years later, my big, fluffy, white dog, Shiloh, came to live with us. One thing this 70 lb. dog does not do is walk on a leash. That didn't really matter as much as I'd thought it did because I got older and simply could no longer deal with the Arizona heat. I wonder if the chemotherapy had anything to do with that.

My third attempt at exercise was with an online app. This one was sort of chair yoga. I hadn't remembered about the bone on bone in my neck or the neuropathy in my hands and feet. Ouch! Not to worry, I'll find something; it's just a matter of trying.

Meanwhile, let's take a look at why it's so important for us to exercise. It's important for everyone, but I mean chronic kidney disease patients and diabetics specifically.

"This is something I explored in my first CKD book: ***What Is It and How Did I Get It? Early Stage Chronic Kidney Disease***:

'I knew exercise was important to control my weight. It would also improve my blood pressure and lower my cholesterol and triglycerides. The greater your triglycerides, the greater the risk of increasing your creatinine. There were other benefits, too, although you didn't have to have CKD to enjoy them: better sleep and improved muscle function and strength. But, as with everything else you do that might impinge upon your health, check with your doctor before you start exercising....

Keeping it simple, basically, there's a compound released by voluntary muscle contraction. It tells the body to repair itself and grow stronger. The idea is to start exercising slowly and then intensify your activity....

What I didn't know at the time is that your body becomes accustomed to a certain kind of exercise and then it isn't as effective anymore....'"

I revisited the topic of exercise towards the end of last year and found new information, which makes sense since more than 10 years have passed since the publication of my first CKD book:

"As for lowering both parts of your blood pressure, that's good news too since high blood pressure is the second most common cause of CKD .... By the way, systolic is the top number which measures your heart rate when blood is being pumped to all parts of your body. Diastolic is the bottom number which measure your heart rate when your heart is at rest.

Lowering your BMI is also a boon. Excess weight may lead to diabetes which, in turn, could lead to CKD. According to the National Center Biotechnology Information [NCBI],

'A high body mass index is one of the strongest risk factors for new-onset CKD. In individuals affected by obesity, a compensatory hyperfiltration occurs to meet the heightened metabolic demands of the increased body weight. The increase in intraglomerular pressure can damage the kidneys and raise the risk of developing CKD in the long term.'"

And then, there's the latest information about exercise from the National Kidney Foundation:

"How does exercise benefit me?

With exercise, it becomes easier to get around, do your necessary tasks and still have some energy left over for other activities you enjoy.

In addition to increased energy, other benefits from exercise may include:

Improved muscle physical functioning

Better blood pressure control

Improved muscle strength

Lowered level of blood fats (cholesterol and triglycerides)

Better sleep

Better control of body weight ….

Type of Exercise

Choose continuous activity such as walking, swimming, bicycling (indoors or out), skiing, aerobic dancing or any other activities in which you need to move large muscle groups continuously.

Low-level strengthening exercises may also be beneficial as part of your program. Design your program to use low weights and high repetitions, and avoid heavy lifting.

How Long to Exercise

Work toward 30 minutes a session. You should build up gradually to this level.

There is nothing magical about 30 minutes. If you feel like walking 45 to 60 minutes, go ahead.

How Often to Exercise

Exercise at least three days a week. These should be non-consecutive days, for example, Monday, Wednesday and Friday. Three days a week is the minimum requirement to achieve the benefits of your exercise.

How Hard to Work While Exercising

This is the most difficult to talk about without knowing your own exercise capacity. Usually, the following ideas are helpful:

Your breathing should not be so hard that you cannot talk with someone exercising with you. (Try to get an exercise partner such as a family member or a friend.) You should feel completely normal within one hour after exercising. (If not, slow down next time.)

You should not feel so much muscle soreness that it keeps you from exercising the next session.

The intensity should be a "comfortable push" level.

Start out slowly each session to warm up, then pick up your pace, then slow down again when you are about to finish.

The most important thing is to start slowly and progress gradually, allowing your body to adapt to the increased levels of activity."

There's more on their website. No excuses now. Let's go exercise.

8/22 *Another New Concept*

Let's see how many of you know this new concept. Well, it's new to me anyway: DUTCH. I'll bet it doesn't ring any bells for you either. I'll give you a hint. It's an acronym, not an adjective. Ugh! I keep forgetting not everyone was an English teacher. An acronym is when you use just the first letters of a phrase rather than spelling each word out. An adjective describes a noun [person, place, thing, or idea].

I gave in and started researching it. Dr. Lisa Watson, a naturopathic doctor from Canada, explains:

"DUTCH is an acronym that stands for Dried Urine Test for Comprehensive Hormones. It is a simple, but sophisticated test that looks not just at your hormones, but how your body processes and metabolizes them.

The DUTCH test looks not just at your reproductive hormones (although it does look at those quite thoroughly), but it also looks at your stress hormones, your androgens (male pattern hormones), your melatonin and the new DUTCH test also looks at organic acids – markers for mood and nutritional balance in the body."

Of course, then I wanted to know what dried urine had to do with it. I found the answer at DUTCH test complete collection instructions:

"Complete all information on each collection device.

 Saturate the filter paper by urinating directly on it OR use a clean cup and dip the filter paper. Leave the collection device open to dry for at least 24 hours.

Once dry, close each collection device. Place all devices in the resealable plastic bag and return in the provided envelope...."

So now we know what it is and how to do it, but what does it have to do with us? The answer may be in what it is that the D.U.T.C.H. looks at. The Holland Clinic [fortunate name for this test information, isn't it?] lists the following hormones:

"Cortisol

Cortisone

Estradiol

Estrone

Estriol

Progesterone

Testosterone

DHEA

Melatonin

This test also measures cortisol and cortisone rhythms and levels, and estrogen metabolism pathways."

Before we get to how any of these affect the kidneys or diabetes, here's a reminder of what hormones are from The Cleveland Clinic:

"Hormones are chemicals that coordinate different functions in your body by carrying messages through your blood to your organs, skin, muscles and other tissues. These signals tell your body what to do and when to do it. Hormones are essential for life and your health."

Cortisone is synthetic cortisol, so let's deal with cortisol.

Does cortisol look familiar? No? Maybe The Mayo Clinic can be helpful here:

"Cortisol, the primary stress hormone, increases sugars (glucose) in the bloodstream, enhances your brain's use of glucose and increases the availability of substances that repair tissues."

Blood sugar or glucose has to do with diabetes. For example, when my NY daughter had a problem and I couldn't go there to help her with it, I had high blood sugar until it was resolved. And what does high blood sugar do to you? I turned to Healthline to see if I could find an answer... and I did:

"If high blood sugar levels go untreated for too long, glucose will build up in your bloodstream and your cells will be starved for fuel. Your cells will use fat for fuel instead.

When your cells use fat instead of glucose, the process produces a byproduct called ketones:

People with diabetes can develop diabetic ketoacidosis (DKA), a potentially deadly condition that causes the blood to become too acidic. Because of poorly functioning insulin in people with diabetes, ketone levels aren't kept in check and can rise to dangerous levels very quickly. DKA can result in diabetic coma or death."

Whoa, baby! How do we recognize this dangerous state before it puts us in a coma or kills us?

"Early symptoms include the following:

Thirst or a very dry mouth

Frequent urination

High blood glucose (blood sugar) levels

High levels of ketones in the urine

Then, other symptoms appear:

Constantly feeling tired

Dry or flushed skin

Nausea, vomiting, or abdominal pain. Vomiting can be caused by many illnesses, not just ketoacidosis. If vomiting continues for more than two hours, contact your health care provider.

Difficulty breathing

Fruity odor on breath

A hard time paying attention, or confusion"

Thank you to Diabetes.org for the above information.

So, is D.U.T.C.H. worth your time, effort, and money? That's between you and your doctor. I do need to let you know I found both nutritionists and endocrinologists online who felt the test was not worth the $119-$600 it costs. It is not covered by insurance. I've also read that they feel this test is useless since other tests can offer the same information in their results. So many pros and cons!

8/29/22 *There is a Difference, You Know*

I usually write the blog on Friday since that's the quietest day of the week in my house. Not this week, though. Bear had doctors' appointments in two different offices. That sort of blew the day for us since we had lunch in-between and I'm just no good after 3:30. My brain and my body seem to shut down then.

More often than not, I don't know what I'm going to write about until I wake up that morning. I have not only the topic in my mind then, but also the opening paragraphs. I hadn't realized how lucky I am to have this sort of, well, magic until I started talking with other writers about it.

Today is all about diabetes. Here's why: Last May, I wrote about CGM or Continuous Glucose Monitor. This sentence is from that blog:

"The fluid mentioned in discussing the CGM is not your hemoglobin, but your blood serum."

I remember being surprised and wondering what the difference was. Today, we find out. How about a few definitions first?

Blood serum - "the clear yellowish fluid that remains from blood plasma after clotting factors (such as fibrinogen and prothrombin) have been removed by clot formation" [Merriam-Webster Dictionary]

Continuous Glucose Monitor - "Continuous glucose monitoring (CGM) devices help you manage Type 1 or Type 2 diabetes with fewer fingerstick tests. A sensor just under your skin measures your glucose levels 24 hours a day. A transmitter sends results to a wearable device or cell phone. It takes time to learn how to use CGM, but it can help you more easily manage your health." [Cleveland Clinic]

Hemoglobin - "Hemoglobin is an iron-rich protein in red blood cells. Oxygen entering the lungs attaches to hemoglobin in the blood, which carries it to tissues in the body."
[MedicalNewsToday]

I like how I got to use my favorite dictionary of all time just now. Back to CGMs. I stumbled across a manufacturer's site that explained quite a bit about CGMs. I am not endorsing the product, but am thankful for Medtronic's explanation:

"Your sensor glucose (SG) readings are taken from your interstitial fluid, and not from your blood, like fingersticks. Interstitial fluid is the fluid that surrounds the cells of your tissue below your skin, and usually glucose moves from your blood vessels and capillaries first and then into When on the rise, the BG value is greater than the SG that follows behind it. But when moving down the tracks, the BG in front is now less than the SG value.

A few points to remember when using CGM with your MiniMed® 530G with Enlite® [Gail here – I'm guessing this holds true for other CMGs, too, since it makes sense.]:

SG and BG readings will rarely match and are expected to be different

A greater difference between SG and BG will be seen when your glucose is changing quickly, such as after eating or after taking a bolus of insulin

And most importantly, always confirm with your BG value before deciding to correct a high or treat a low glucose

Here's A Tip: Knowing the direction and speed of your glucose changes will be more useful than focusing on individual BG or sensor readings. When using continuous glucose monitoring (CGM) trends are the key. In fact, seeing trends and patterns in your glucose is likely one of the primary reasons you started using CGM therapy. Trends highlight the direction that your sensor glucose readings are moving and the speed at which they are changing. Fingerstick blood glucose readings and sensor glucose readings are only snapshots of your glucose at that very moment. Trends can tell you if your glucose has been rising, falling, or appears to have been stable over several minutes, hours, and even the day.

So it's important not to focus too much on the individual sensor glucose numbers (as it is likely to be different from your BG meter reading) and more on trends and patterns in your glucose levels."

NewsMedicalLifeSciences has an interesting bit of information for us:

"Whole blood and serum blood glucose is often different. Red blood cells have higher concentration of protein than serum and serum has higher water content and more dissolved glucose than whole blood. To obtain blood glucose in serum from figures in whole blood, it is multiplied by 1.15."

Between pre-diabetes and diabetes type 2, I've been in the diabetes world for years. Yet, no one – nephrologist, PCP, nor endocrinologist – has ever mentioned this to me. You'd think at least the endocrinologist would.

I also find it interesting that I'd never been told about the 5-10 minute delay in accurately reporting serum blood glucose. What 5-10 minute delay, you ask. Whoops, I neglected to explain it, didn't I? No problem. ResearchGate can do that for us:

"This delay is the consequence of the process of glucose diffusion across the walls of capillary vessels and through the interstitial space to the sensor. This process requires some time, and the delay can be observed during both rising and decreasing BG values, probably with varying impact."

The National Institutes of Health offer a succinct summary of the advantages and disadvantages of serum blood glucose testing:

"Advantages: In patients requiring insulin therapy (both type 1 diabetes and in patients with type 2 diabetes requiring intensive insulin therapy and or sulfonylureas, flash monitoring has been demonstrated to be cost-effective when compared to CBG self-monitoring of blood glucose (SMBG). Interstitial glucose measurements are recorded as frequently as every 5 minutes every hour, which has the benefit of monitoring for hypoglycemia during sleep at night.

Disadvantages: Glucose is first seen in blood before it is seen in the interstitial fluid, which the CGM measures hence may not always be a reliable indicator in rapidly changing blood glucose levels. The high cost of sensors and machines (approximately $5000 per annum) may not make this a viable option in economically less advantaged clients and communities where health care is not subsidized by insurance or the government."

As for me, I'm glad not to have those finger pricks anymore. I'm only human, after all.

9/5 That Delicious All-American Italian Food: Pizza

Last night, my grandson had pizza for dinner along with his vegetables and fruit. We were facetiming with him during his dinner. So, then Bear wanted pizza for dinner. I hesitated. Wasn't even good pizza junk food? And, therefore, not on the renal diet? Why isn't it, I wondered because I like pizza, too.

Verywellfit, a nutrition and exercise site, offers the following information about one slice of pizza:

"The following nutrition information is provided by the U.S. Department of Agriculture (USDA) for one slice (107g) of regular cheese pizza from a standard fast-food pizza chain...

Calories: 285

Fat: 10.4g

Sodium: 640mg

Carbohydrates: 35.6g

Fiber: 2.5g

Sugars: 3.8g

Protein: 12.2g"

Since we are chronic kidney disease patients, let's start with the obvious. Yes, sodium. The Ontario Renal Network suggests 2000 mg. of sodium a day for us, but also suggests we speak with our nephrologists or dietitians for a more specific individualized number. For example, men are often permitted more sodium since they have larger bodies. But that, too, is a generalization.

I don't know about you, but I find it hard to eat only one slice of pizza. Two slices have 1,280 mg. of sodium. That's already 60% of my sodium intake! Don't forget I'll be eating two other meals, a bedtime snack [I'm a diabetic] and have sides with my pizza.

And protein? What about protein? The usual limitation for chronic kidney disease patients is five ounces. Again, this is a generalization. Your nephrologist or dietitian will be able to individualize the amount of protein you can safely have each day. Five ounces equals about 141,748 grams. Two slices of pizza – plain, cheese pizza – only has 24.4 grams of protein. But how many of you eat plain, cheese pizza? Bear adds meatballs, ham, bacon, Italian sausage, and pepperoni [No, I don't eat any slices from his half.]. Add up the grams of protein. I'm pretty sure the add ons will either wipe out or greatly reduce the amount of protein you can have in your other meals the day you have pizza.

As a diabetic, I need to limit my lunch and dinner carbohydrate intake to 45 grams per meal. Two slices of pizza equal a carbohydrate intake of 71.2 grams. Since the main thrust of the diabetes diet is to keep your blood sugar on a steady level, going that far over my carbohydrate limit for lunch or dinner is going to cause a blood glucose spike. For those of you who like cold pizza for breakfast [Who? Me?], the diabetic carbohydrate limit for breakfast is 30 grams. Even if you have only one slice, you're already over your breakfast limit for carbohydrates.

I don't even want to start on sugar intake as a diabetic. In and of itself, the 7.6 grams of sugar in two slices of pizza is not necessarily a problem except that again - you have to eat two other meals and a snack. They, also, are going to contain sugar and you probably don't know how much until you decide what to eat for that particular meal. Let's remember what the Nation Kidney Foundation has to say about diabetes:

"Over time, having high blood sugar from diabetes can cause damage inside your kidneys. As a result, they filter out some good things along with waste. As more damage happens, kidneys will have less function and waste builds up."

For those of you without diabetes or CKD, diabetes is the leading cause of CKD. Avoid it by all means.

I would say the fiber is a good thing. It seems most of us don't eat enough fiber. Too little fiber may lead to constipation. As DaVita puts it:

"Many people with CKD don't get enough fiber because many fiber sources are too high in potassium and phosphorus [Gail here: These are two electrolytes that are also limited on the renal diet]. Increasing your fiber intake, [sic] can cause gas, bloating and cramps."

DaVita, a CKD education and dialysis company, has a good list of foods that both contain fiber and are on the kidney diet.

As for fat, I wasn't too sure about what role that plays in your diet, so I turned to the American Kidney Fund for help:

"Fat gives you energy and helps you use some of the vitamins in your food. You need some fat in your eating plan to stay healthy. Too much fat can lead to weight gain and heart disease. Limit fat in your meal plan, and choose healthier fats when you can, such as olive oil."

But then there's more on the plus side of fat:

"When we first look at a pizza, it might appear to be high in fat content. Again, research has shown that the fat content of most pizza rarely exceeds the 10% level. Compare this to a piece of steak with upwards of 20% fat, and you begin to realize just how good pizza really is. On top of all this, because vegetable oil, olive oil, and oil-based shortenings are commonly used in the crust formulation, pizza and pizza products (calzone, stromboli, and bread sticks) are good sources of polyunsaturated fat, with only modest cholesterol contributions (through meat and cheese toppings) to the diet."

Thank you to PMA Pizza Media, a pizza trade vehicle, for the above information.

And finally, the caloric intake, which is a whopping 570 calories [about 46 minutes of running for goodness sake!] for two slices. Your calorie intake limitation for CKD is highly individualized, so let's make things easy and use my 1350 to 1450 restriction. Should I eat those two slices of delicious cheese pizza [which would really be a vegetable pizza for me raising the number of calories even more], I have just eaten almost half of my caloric intake for the day. Do I – or you – really love pizza that much? I have to admit I do, although I don't have pizza too often.

This was fun, taking pizza apart and then putting it back together again. I suspect you'll find another blog dealing with what is usually considered sort of a junk food soon. I've got to admit I'm not so sure this is a junk food anymore.

9/12 **What a Waste**

Once again, my online friend Geo mentioned something related to chronic kidney disease that I hadn't thought of. His point of view about chronic kidney disease is a lot different than mine. When Geo brings something to my attention, he also includes medical links. I read them and thought to myself, "Thanks, Geo. This is something CKD patients should know about."

The something is Hydroxymethylbutyrate. That's quite a mouthful, so it's usually referred to as HMB. Ring any bells? It didn't for me, so I turned to WebMD to find out just what this is.

"Hydroxymethylbutyrate (HMB) is a chemical that is produced when the body breaks down leucine. Leucine is an amino acid, one of the building blocks of protein. People use HMB to make medicine.
[Gail here: I thought that might be a typo, but no, that's the quote.]

HMB is most commonly used for building muscle or preventing muscle loss."

Apparently, it many different names according to the same source:

"Beta-hydroxy-beta-methylbutyrate, B-Hydroxy B-Methylbutyrate Monohydreate, Beta-Hydroxy-Beta-Methylbutyric Acid, Calcium B-Hydroxy B-Methylbutyrate Monohydrate, Calcium HMB, Hidroximetilbutirato, HMB, HMB de Calcium, Hydroxyméthylbutyrate, Hydroxymethyl Butyrate, Hydroxyethyl Butyrate"

Hmm, so what does preventing muscle loss have to do with us? I imagine body builders might also use it to build muscle. That, of course, is pure conjecture on my part. Wait a minute, I do remember something about muscle loss with kidney disease. Maybe that's the angle we should research here. Let's see.

An article in the September 2020 issue of Journal of Nephrology makes it clear just how much this should matter to us.

"Muscle loss is a frequent finding in CKD, especially for patients with more advanced stages of the disease including ESKD patients undergoing hemodialysis (HD) .... The consequences of muscle loss are not only related to physical disability as commonly observed in the elderly. [Gail again: Uh-oh, since the definition of elderly is over 65, this means me... and possibly you.] In fact, many studies in the past decades have also linked muscle loss in CKD patients with worse QoL, depression, PEW, fracture risk, cardiovascular complications, graft failure and post-operative complications in transplant recipients, as well as with increased hospitalization and mortality."

You may need these definitions. I know I did. QoL means quality of life, while PEW means protein energy wasting.

Holy cow! How did I not know this? How does muscle loss work anyway? This explanation is from Nephrology, Dialysis, Transplantation:

"Muscle mass is maintained by the balance of protein metabolism, and small but persistent imbalances between protein synthesis [That means one of the most fundamental biological processes by which individual cells build their specific proteins.] and degradation will induce muscle wasting. It is now recognized that the catabolic [Catabolism is the part of the metabolism responsible for breaking complex molecules down into smaller molecules.] environment of CKD, which includes metabolic acidosis [the buildup of acid in the body due to kidney disease or kidney failure], inflammation, increased glucocorticoid [a kind of steroid] production and suppressed insulin/insulin-like growth factor 1

(IGF-1) signalling [sic] stimulates and accelerates substantial muscle protein loss through the activation of protein degradation, suppression of protein synthesis and impairment of muscle regeneration ...."

Sorry about all the inserts, but definitions were needed. Thanks to all the different dictionaries that afforded these definitions. Anyway, this does not sound good, folks. Maybe we'd better find out how we can recognize this in ourselves.

It's a little bit technical, but the out-take from this year's Nutritional Management of Renal Disease (Fourth Edition) on Science Direct offers the answer we're looking for:

"PEW is manifested by low levels of serum albumin or prealbumin, sarcopenia [a condition characterized by loss of muscle mass], weight loss, vascular calcification, and increased levels of C-reactive protein, and it is closely associated with increased risk of morbidity and mortality and impaired quality of life...."

No good. We have to do something about this, but what? The most usual answer I found as I scoured website after website is Krager's Blood Purification study:

"We have reviewed the pathophysiology of pertinent nutritional issues across the CKD, ESRD, and transplant CKD spectrum. New developments include nutritional benefits of intradialytic meal replacement, scoring systems for PEW, and the emerging field of exercise therapy in CKD and ESRD to combat frailty and reverse the effects of PEW."

I'm sorry, Geo, I could find very little about using HMB to treat protein wasting in CKD. The good news is that it does no harm to the kidneys, either. Every website I pulled up made that conclusion. More good news is that,

"HMB is an effective supplement for those who want to speed up their recovery from high-intensity exercise — both weight training and endurance cardio. It helps to boost and preserve muscle mass and strength, and can be useful for weight loss...."

The above quote is from MyProtein, a training site that does sell supplements. However, it was written by a registered dietitian.

Let's get back to what CKD patients can do for protein wasting now. PubMed Central recommends the following:

- Dietary Intervention
- Phosphorus management
- Alkali therapy for metabolic acidosis
- Exercise

This was a hard blog to write. The ones with concepts that are new to me usually are. But I thoroughly enjoy learning about new concepts, so I don't mind how hard it was. I hope you learned something new, too.

Topic change: These are the CDC's statistics as of last year,

"More than 1 in 7, that is 15% of US adults or 37 million people, are estimated to have CKD. As many as 9 in 10 adults with CKD do not know they have CKD. About 2 in 5 adults with severe CKD do not know they have CKD."

You know what to do: urge your friends and family to take the simple blood and urine tests for CKD.

9/19 Meet Me at the Meeting

I registered for my second Association of American Kidney Patients Annual National Patient Meeting. This was their 47th. My first was several years ago in Tampa, Florida. I was thrilled to see other chronic kidney disease awareness advocates I'd been working with and meet new ones. Due to Covid, I don't attend live meetings anymore. This year's AAKP meeting was virtual... just my style these days.

It occurred to me that I hadn't blogged about AAKP in a while. It's time, isn't it? I've long been fascinated by how this organization started as grass roots operation. This is from AAKP's About Us page:

"The American Association of Kidney Patients (AAKP) is the oldest and largest fully independent kidney patient organization in the U.S. Founded in 1969 by six dialysis patients, with doctor encouragement, our Founders helped create the End Stage Renal Disease (ESRD) Program, saving more than one million lives since 1973.

Founded by Patients for Patients

Our Founders wanted to form an organization that would elevate the kidney patient voice in the national healthcare arena, provide patients with educational resources to improve their lives, and give kidney patients and their family members a sense of community. These patients met twice a week in the King's County hospital ward (NY) and while hooked up to primitive dialysis machines for 12 to 18 hours at a time they brainstormed, researched and eventually formed AAKP.

The group originally called themselves NAPH (National Association of Patients on Hemodialysis, which later changed to AAKP) ...."

Fascinating, isn't it? Before we go any further, I want to make certain you understand that this is not an advertisement, nor am I selling you anything. Membership and the meeting are both free.

What goes on at these meetings, you might be wondering. This year, the meeting was from September 21-23 and offered so many different educational opportunities. We know I'm not on dialysis and am stage 3B. There were plenty of outbreak sessions I was interested in. Some of these were:

"Disease Management: Lab Values Explained! The Importance of Knowing Your Numbers & What Those Numbers May Mean for Your Health This session is proudly sponsored by CareDx, Inc. Lana Schmidt, AAKP National Board of Director, Ambassador, former dialysis patient, current transplant recipient Prabir Roy-Chaudhury, MD, PhD, FRCP (Edin); Professor of Medicine and Co-Director of the University of North Carolina (UNC) Kidney Center

Disease Management: Be Prepared: What Kidney Patients Should Know Before Going into the Hospital This session is proudly sponsored by AstraZeneca. Leigh-Ann Williams, AAKP Ambassador, home hemodialysis patient Rohan S. Paul, MBBS, transplant nephrologist with Washington University in St. Louis, and the George Washington Transplant Institute; Member, Public Policy Committee, American Society of Transplantation (AST)

Disease Management: Staying Healthy with Kidney Disease This session is proudly sponsored by Otsuka Pharmaceuticals. Jim Myers, AAKP National Board of Director, Ambassador, former dialysis patient, current transplant recipient Stephen Fadem, MD, FACP, FASN; Chair, AAKP Medical Advisory Board; Clinical Professor of Medicine, Baylor College of Medicine, Section of Nephrology"

Should you be preparing for a transplant, transplanted already, or on dialysis, there were plenty of outbreak sessions for you, too. Everyone was covered in this meeting. Then there were the outbreak sessions about spreading awareness, research and innovation. You name it, there was probably an outbreak session for it.

Of course, there were also approximately hour-long general sessions on such topics as diversity, xenotransplantation, books as awareness [shoutout to Suzanne Ruff and Risa Simon], and even the need for a kidney emoji – no kidding.

Lest you think this was all too intense [well, except for the emoji general session - although that's a more serious topic than you suspect.], there were sponsor halls to view and networking conversations to join. There was even a five minute "wellness" break during the day. I wonder if that means bathroom or water break.

I don't think I've mentioned the breakout sessions for vets or on the kidney diet yet. They were very helpful for those vets who were unaware of the kidney diet. I'm saying this because I just got an email from a vet whose doctor told him to just watch his sodium intake. The vet is at stage 3A and felt he could be doing more to prevent his CKD from progressing quickly. He was right.

By the way, this year's meeting theme was "Patient Consumers: Leaders for Kidney Research and Innovation." We are the patient consumers – you and me. It follows that we are then the leaders in research and innovation. In order to fulfill that role, we need to educate ourselves about our kidneys, our conditions [stage, dialysis, transplant], how we can better our conditions, and how to get the word out for kidney disease awareness. We also need to know what innovations are on the horizon and how we can help our government help us. It sounds like a tall order, but the meeting helped those attending learn whatever they choose to.

So, how do you get to go to next year's marvelous meeting [Oh goody, alliteration]? You can register directly on AAKP's website. Those of you reading the blog on your computers can click through. On their website, you can also view the annual patient meetings of the last three years via YouTube to get an idea of what it's like. You should also know that the meeting is interactive. Should you decide to register, you do need a computer and either Chrome or Foxfire.

9/26 *Life Long Learning*

The American Association of Kidney Patients' 47th Annual National Meeting concluded last Friday. The first time I attended, before cancer and Covid, it was in person. I wondered how this year's online meeting would go. Would I learn anything new? Could I interact with others? Would there be people there I already knew?

The answer to each of these questions is yes. What I think would most interest you is what I learned. I've heard of PCORI years ago when I first started working as a pharmaceutical patient advisor. It was mentioned to me just before a session started and not brought up again during the meeting. Since I was there to offer my suggestions, not learn about any other organizations, I didn't pursue it.

PCORI stands for Patient-Centered Outcomes Research Institute. It's also fairly new since it was created in 2010 [two years after I was diagnosed with CKD]. I found the following on their website and thought it clearly explains who they are:

"PCORI'S STRATEGIC PLAN Highlights for Patients, Caregivers, and Patient Advocates

PCORI'S STRATEGIC PLAN

Generating Evidence to Achieve More Efficient, Effective, and Equitable Health Care and Improve Health for All

Strategic Plan builds on our past work and outlines a bold approach to addressing the challenges that a changing health and healthcare system poses to the people we serve.

Our National Priorities for Health focus on improving health outcomes and patient care through research and other programs. Their connected nature will allow PCORI to continue to fund research and other programs to improve patient care and health outcomes.

NATIONAL PRIORITIES FOR HEALTH

Increase Evidence for Existing Interventions and Emerging Innovations in Health

Enhance Infrastructure to Accelerate Patient Centered Outcomes Research

Advance the Science of Dissemination, Implementation, and Health Communication

Achieve Health Equity

Accelerate Progress Toward an Integrated Learning Health System

A HOLISTIC APPROACH

The core parts work together to drive our mission. PCORI will track and measure our efforts so we can make improvements along the way.

Promoting Engagement

Creating a culture that is inclusive through meaningful engagement with patients, caregivers, and other stakeholders across all aspects of research.

Funding Patient-Centered CER

Funding comparative clinical effectiveness research, CER, that puts patients at the center. This means funding research that answers questions important to patients and others. Our Research Agenda, made up of six broad areas of research, provides the framework for this effort.

Strengthening Key Infrastructure

Advancing the science and methods of CER and developing the workforce, data and tools that can make research and delivery of care more patient centric.

Sharing and Using Research Findings

Investing in the science and practice of helping to make sure results from our PCORI-funded studies are easy to find and are more widely used to make better healthcare choices.

ENHANCED FOCUS ON

EQUITY

Health equity is woven through our National Priorities for Health and our Research Agenda. This expands on our commitment to health equity in all that we do and includes:

• Sharpening our focus on generating evidence with a direct impact on improving patient centered care, health outcomes, and a person's overall health status.

• Partnering with the communities we serve and that make our work possible.

PRIORITIZING MATERNAL

HEALTH AND INTELLECTUAL AND

DEVELOPMENTAL DISABILITIES

We are committed to research focused on improving health outcomes for:

• Pregnant people, mainly at high-risk periods before, during, and after childbirth.

• People with intellectual and developmental disabilities, and those who care for them as infants and into adulthood."

I thought this whole concept was spectacular, but what did it have to do with chronic kidney disease? Or any kind of kidney disease for that matter.

Hmmm, it seems they conducted a study of depression while on dialysis which contrasted two different anti-depression medications:

"A PCORI-funded study found that CBT improved depression about as much as sertraline for patients on dialysis with depression. The research team found improvements across all patients in sleep, appetite, mood, energy level, and ability to focus. At the end of the study, about a third of all patients no longer had symptoms of depression.

Compared with patients using CBT, patients taking sertraline had slightly more improvement in symptoms of depression. But patients taking sertraline also had side effects more often than patients using CBT."

PCORI also answered the following question with research:

"Does an Online Decision Aid Help People with Advanced Chronic Kidney Disease Choose between Two Treatment Options? [hemodialysis and peritoneal dialysis]

The decision aid increased

What patients knew about CKD and treatment options

How sure patients were about what was most important to them in choosing between treatments

How sure patients felt about which treatment they would choose

The decision aid didn't change patients' self-confidence in their ability to decide which treatment would be best for them."

In a still ongoing study, "the research team is comparing ways to monitor and treat high blood pressure in children with CKD."

PCORI also deals with diabetes, the number one cause of CKD. This is the conclusion of the study:

"Comparing Three Methods to Help Patients Manage Type 2 Diabetes

Our project demonstrated that C4L and community health workers, alone and in combination, improve self-management skills and control of DM [Diabetes Meliltus] in an inner-city Medicaid population to a similar extent. Both C4L and CHWs integrated into a medical team activate and sustain patient engagement in DM care, promoting achievement of wellness and clinical goals, reducing HbA1c, and lowering health care utilization. CHWs support patients with DM by addressing both medical needs and the social determinants of chronic disease. In addition, CHWs may enhance patient engagement with mHealth by acting as digital navigators. In the future, a potential combination strategy may start by providing patients with a CHW and transitioning to mHealth support, with reintroduction of CHWs as needed to maintain patient healthy behaviors."

If you're anything like me, you'll need more information about C4L from the same source:

"The key features of the C4L system can be accessed via secure text messaging and can be used on any cell phone handset. C4L features include the following: (1) reminders to check glucose and Blood pressure; (2) recording and transmission of physiologic parameters (glucose, BP) with alarms set by the health care team for specified critical values that are sent to the patient; (3) reminders to take medications; (4) tracking of lifestyle and behavioral goals using selected questionnaires; (5) summary reports for the patient and health care provider; and (6) educational and lifestyle modification tips to educate and support self-care skills."

All I have to say is, "Many thanks to you, PCORI."

10/3 aHus is …

When I first stumbled upon this word, I thought it might have something to do with marriage since the initial syllable of husband is hus. According to Vocabulary.com,

"The word husband comes from the Old Norse hūsbōndi, where hūs meant house and bōndi meant dweller."

But then, I looked up aHus. Was I ever wrong in assuming this had to do with a house. I turned to my trusted favorites to see what I could find out about this word I hadn't heard before, starting with the American Kidney Fund:

"aHUS (atypical hemolytic uremic syndrome) is a very rare disease that causes tiny blood clots to form in the small blood vessels of your body. These blood clots can block blood flow to important organs, such as your kidneys. This can damage your kidneys and lead to kidney failure."

I'm pretty sure we all know what atypical and syndrome mean. Just in case you forgot, uremic means of or about the urine. And hemolytic? That means blood (hemo) and lysis (rupturing). Or in this case,

"rupturing of the red blood cells and the release of their contents into the surrounding fluid."

Thanks for helping us out here, Wikipedia. While this was the most reader friendly definition I could find, keep in mind that anyone can edit a Wikipedia entry.

So, we're back in the realm of rare diseases. I'd like to know what causes this particular rare disease. Since it is a rare disease, I went to GARD's website for information about how one gets this disease. By the way, GARD is the new website for Genetic and Rare Diseases and is part of National Center for Advancing Translational Sciences. That's part of the U.S. Department of Health and Human Services' National Institutes of Health.

"It can occur at any age and is often caused by a combination of environmental and genetic factors. Genetic factors involve genes that code for proteins that help control the complement system (part of your body's immune system). Environmental factors include certain medications (such as anticancer drugs), chronic diseases (e.g., systemic sclerosis and malignant hypertension), viral or bacterial infections, cancers, organ transplantation, and pregnancy. In about 60% of aHUS, a genetic change may be identified. The genes associated with genetic aHUS include C3, CD46 (MCP), CFB, CFH, CFHR1, CFHR3, CFHR4, CFI, DGKE, and THBD. Genetic changes in these genes increase the likelihood (predisposition) to developing aHUS, rather than directly causing the disease. In most cases, there is no family history of the disease. In cases that do run in families, predisposition to aHUS is inherited in an autosomal dominant or an autosomal recessive pattern of inheritance."

Uh-oh, did you notice 'organ transplantation' as one of the environmental factors which may cause this disease? And 'chronic disease'? That makes it even more important for us to know how to recognize if we have this disease. Well, how do we do that?

I went to the site called aHusNews to see if they could pinpoint the symptoms. Sure enough, they could.

"Often, people with aHUS will report a vague feeling of illness, with non-specific symptoms that may include paleness, nausea, vomiting, fatigue, drowsiness, high blood pressure, and swelling.

There are three hallmark symptoms that define aHUS: hemolytic anemia, thrombocytopenia, and kidney failure.

Symptoms can appear at any age, though it is slightly more common for them to first appear in childhood rather than later on in life. Adult-onset aHUS is more frequent in biological females than males, whereas childhood-onset disease affects both sexes equally."

Is that how it's diagnosed, I wondered. A different site, called Ahus.org was helpful here.

"…. After initial blood tests, the hospital may conduct Creatinine and BUN tests and may (or may not) reach an initial Diagnosis of atypical HUS. The flu like symptoms … will continue to worsen when episodes are active. At this point, kidney function may begin to fall, often quite dramatically. Other organs sometime experience problems in some cases. Quite often, seizures have been reported, along with other neurological issues. Sometimes gastronomical problems occur as well.

During an extended atypical attack or episode, the tell-tale signs of aHUS are very obvious. Hemoglobin levels may fall to 6-7, when normal levels should be 11-13: Hematocrit levels may fall in the low 20s, when normal levels should be in the mid 30s. Creatinine and BUN levels start to rise, characteristics of failing kidney function. Blood Pressure will become a nagging, recurring problem. Diarrhea and vomiting may also be present (sometimes that occurs with the initial onset, at other times it occurs later) ….

TRIGGERS VS. THE CAUSE

It is important not to confuse 'triggers' of atypical HUS with the root cause. In normal life, many of us get colds, the flu, infections, and the body's immune system deal with those properly. In aHUS, a person may get a cold, and it triggers a full blown aHUS episode. This occurs simply because the body's immune system is not reacting properly to the event."

The site mentions other specific tests that may be done to diagnose aHus.

All this is worrisome. Is there, perhaps, a cure? No, there isn't. This is a lifelong disease, but there are treatments available. Our old friend WebMD explains:

"The FDA has approved two drugs to treat aHUS:

Eculizumab (Soliris)

Ravulizumab (Ultomirus)

Both drugs are monoclonal antibodies. These are human-made proteins that act like natural antibody proteins in your body. They attach to other proteins called antigens. Once they attach, they tell your immune system to destroy cells with that antigen.

Eculizumab can increase your blood platelet and red blood cell counts. If you take it early enough, it can also reverse any kidney damage you have.

Your doctor will give you eculizumab by injection in their office. You may have side effects from the drug…. You can also get ravulizumab as an injection. Common side effects include high blood pressure, headache, and cold symptoms. You could also have digestive system problems such as diarrhea, nausea, and vomiting.

Eculizumab and ravulizumab are a type of drug called complement inhibitors. These kinds of drugs may carry a risk of getting meningococcal disease. The CDC suggests people taking them get a meningococcal vaccine. Your doctor may also suggest you take antibiotics to help prevent meningococcal disease.

Besides eculizumab and ravulizumab, you can also treat the symptoms of aHUS with plasma therapy. Plasma is a liquid portion of your blood that takes important nutrients, hormones, and proteins throughout your body.

When you get plasma therapy, you may either have a plasma infusion or plasma exchange.

In a plasma infusion, a doctor puts plasma from a donor into your body. In a plasma exchange, a doctor filters plasma parts out of your blood and replaces them with donor plasma.

If your kidneys don't respond to treatment, you may need kidney dialysis or a kidney transplant."

Now you know whether you wanted to or not. I'm sorry.

10/10 **NORD**

Last week, I wrote about a rare kidney disease: aHus. I also wrote about the National Organization for Rare Disorders [NORD]. I questioned whether people who may need their services really know about NORD. Here comes the famous 'just in case.' Just in case you are one of these patients, allow me to introduce you to NORD. According to their website:

"If you live with a rare disease, or love someone who does, NORD is here to help you. For more than 30 years, we have been providing services for patients and their families, rare disease patient organizations, medical professionals, and those seeking to develop new diagnostics and treatments. We are here to support every member of the rare disease community with programs and services focused on one ultimate goal: to improve the lives of individuals and families affected by rare diseases."

I can just see you now thinking to yourself, just what are the rare kidney diseases? The National Kidney Foundation was kind enough to list many of them for us:

- "Acute Kidney Injury
- Alport Syndrome
- Nephropathic Cystinosis
- Cystinuria
- Fabry Disease
- Focal Segmental Glomerular Sclerosis (FSGS)
- Membranous Nephropathy
- IgA Nephropathy
- Nephrotic Syndrome

- Polycystic Kidney Disease
- Refractory Gout
- Complement 3 Glomerulopathy (C3G)
- distal Renal Tubular Acidosis (dRTA)"

What's that? Where's aHus, you ask. This list is not complete, but it does give you an idea of how many rare diseases of the kidneys you may not have heard of before. While I've written about some of these, others are brand new to me, too. Today is not a day about a specific disease. Today is NORD's day.

I was curious as to what NORD has to offer those with a rare kidney disease. My kidney disease awareness buddy, Uncle Jim [James Myers] is often in Washington to advocate for us as kidney patients. Since 1983, so have representatives of NORD. In addition, they advocate on the state and local levels. Their advocacy is to ensure policy reflects the needs of these patients. My favorite part of NORD's offerings is their educational program. Patients, their families, friends, and others in their lives are offered education about whichever rare disease they have. Doctors and others in the medical profession are also offered educational about specific rare diseases.

What struck me as being so necessary is covered here, too. I felt it was important to explain their Patient Assistance Program correctly since it seems quite generous that I went right back to their website for a quote:

"NORD pioneered Patient Assistance Programs in 1987 and we are the leader in patient-focused PAPs today. NORD programs include free drug, co-pay and premium assistance, travel/lodging assistance for clinical trials, and expanded or emergency access."

Considering the price of drugs today, although President Biden is doing all he can as fast as he can, this is important. The co-pay and premium assistance are right up there in importance.

NORD mentors patient organizations. I was impressed with their easily understood, comprehensive explanation so we'll go back to their website for that, too:

"Disease-specific patient organizations are crucial partners in our mission to serve rare disease patients and their families. We provide capacity building and mentorship services to start-up and established organizations through one-on-one guidance, webinars, in-person meetings, and toolkits to help them establish, strengthen and grow."

This organization doesn't miss a beat; it also supplies research grants. So far, at least two FDA approved medications have been discovered via these grants. It's through these grants that more information about rare diseases is being discovered.

This national organization has partnerships with the European Organization for Rare Diseases (EURORDIS) and the Japanese Patient Association (JPA). Not only that, but

"NORD represents the U.S. on both Rare Diseases International (RDI) and Rare Disease Day steering committees."

Amazing how much NORD does and, if you're anything like me, you never heard of it until you needed it. On their website, you'll find 65 different rare diseases explained and even videos for Patients & Caregivers, Research & Science, Advocacy, and Medical Education. I took a peek at the Patient & Caregivers' titles. While there were videos on gene editing and other interesting topics, I chose to go to 'New Patients'. There I found nine pages of videos listed, some in Spanish.

I haven't yet mentioned the patient registries where you can enter your information and share your experiences with others around the world. You can learn from their experiences as well. All this information is helpful to research. The FDA, NIH, organizations, and experts are involved as well. You can even start your own registry if there isn't one for your rare disease. Here's the email address for registries: registryinquiry@rarediseases.org. This program is called IAMRARE.

NORD offers links to a number of resources, both internal and external. If you think I admire NORD for all they offer to those with rare diseases, kidney or otherwise, you are correct. You have to remember that I'm not a doctor, so new information I bring to you is often new to me, too.

I do urge you to explore their website. There are free webinars listed on their website, as well as the other sources of information. If I understood the information correctly, membership is open to organizations rather than individuals. I did see a registration category for Advocates.

Enjoy exploring this wonderful website even if you don't have a rare kidney disease or any other kind of rare disease. The learning opportunities are vast.

10/17 *Old vs New*

Some of my friends and family are mixed race. Or, at least, that's what they call themselves. Usually, neither of us cares what they're called. I used to think it was only important in diagnosing and staging chronic kidney disease. I'd been told Blacks have higher muscle mass and that's why they needed their own classification for CKD testing. Not being a doctor [and not really understanding], I accepted that. But where did that leave my mixed-race friends and family, I wondered. The choices were Black or non-Black. They weren't either.

It did seem weird. Maybe we need to know what creatinine has to do with muscle mass. I turned to the Biron Health Group in Canada for a clear explanation:

"Creatinine is a normal product of muscle metabolism (breakdown) and is eliminated through the urine. The level of creatinine in the blood depends on a person's muscle mass and the quality of their renal (kidney) function. Calculation of the estimated glomerular filtration rate (eGFR) allows for variations in people's muscle mass to be taken into account when evaluating their kidney function."

Let's backtrack just a bit here for a definition of eGFR. The 'e' stands for estimated, rather than measured. Measured GFR would have an 'm' before the 'GFR' rather than an 'e.' It's also a more complicated test. GFR is Glomerular Filtration Rate. The National Institutes of Health's National Library of Medicine's MedlinePlus [What a mouthful!] tells us:

"A glomerular filtration rate (GFR) is a blood test that checks how well your kidneys are working. Your kidneys have tiny filters called glomeruli. These filters help remove waste and excess fluid from the blood. A GFR test estimates how much blood passes through these filters each minute."

Okay, let's go back to my mixed race friends and family. It seems I wasn't the only one who had questions. According to the American Kidney Fund:

"A task force led by the National Kidney Foundation (NKF) and the American Society of Nephrology (ASN) was formed in 2020 to look into the use of race in the GFR test. The NKF-ASN Task Force asked patients, the community and kidney disease experts, including AKF's Medical Advisory Committee, to give advice on how to reduce bias in the equations that estimate how well kidneys work. In September 2021, the NKF-ASN Task Force announced recommendations to remove Black race in the eGFR calculation."

Wait a minute. Does that mean that my mixed race friends and family who previously chose the Black or Afro-American classification to calculate their GFR would now have a higher or lower GFR? This is confusing to patients at best. But it doesn't have to be. Let's take a look at the differences.

University of California –Davis Health goes right to the heart of the matter [the kidney of the matter is more like it]:

"Our data showed that a large number of patients in higher risk groups would either be reassigned from stage 3 to stage 4 CKD, or reassigned from CKD-negative to CKD-positive, simply by removing the race parameter from the calculation of their eGFR." Think about that for a minute. It basically means that more people will be treated as they need to be instead of not being treated because they have higher muscle mass as a race. Here's why I am intrigued that the American Medical Association has this insight: "'By acknowledging that race is a social construct and not an inherent risk factor for disease, we can truly make progress toward our goal of attaining health equity for all patients. The AMA will continue to strongly support policies and regulations aimed at eliminating barriers to care and protecting the health of our nation's most vulnerable populations," said Dr. Suk."

Dr. Suk is an AMA Board Member, M.D., J.D., M.P.H. [Master of Public Health], M.B.A.

I wondered how else my mixed race friends and family who identified as Black would now benefit from the GFR calculation without racial classification. Thank you to the National Center for Biotechnology Center for this information:

"Removal of race adjustment may increase CKD diagnoses among Black adults and enhance access to specialist care, medical nutrition therapy, kidney disease education, and kidney transplantation, while potentially excluding kidney donors and prompting drug contraindications or dose reductions for individuals reclassified to advanced stages of CKD. This potential for benefits and harms must be interpreted in light of persistent disparities in care... documented biases of eGFRcr without race... and the historical misuse of race as a biological variable to further racism...."

However, the same source has several warnings for us:

"First, many institutions use the Modification of Diet in Renal Disease (MDRD) equation. Removal of the larger race coefficient in the MDRD (1.212 vs 1.159 in CKD-EPI) would lead to larger decreases in eGFR and more individuals crossing relevant thresholds. Second, some institutions have removed race using methods other than universalizing the "White/other" equation. Third, eGFR does not determine care for all patients. Clinical judgment... unbiased confirmatory tests to corroborate eGFRcr, and varying adherence to guidelines may all influence how changes materialize."

In other words, this is not the universal equation for calculating GFR. It's a step in the right direction, but there's still more work to be done. Monica Hahn, MD, MPH, MS, AAHIVS [American Academy of HIV Medicine] via Practice Update affirms the work that has been done so far:

"…. A recent study found that the removal of the race correction factor and subsequent re-staging of chronic kidney disease would make 14,000 Black patients newly eligible for kidney transplants, and 60,000 newly eligible for specialist referral."

10/24 *Asians Too*

Last week, I wrote about omitting the category 'Afro-American' from the eGFR equation. I thought that was the only issue with the eGFR. You can imagine my surprise when a reader contacted me to tell me her nephrologist won't use the eGFR to stage her chronic kidney disease because she is Asian.

Of course, I felt obliged to research the why of this for her, which means for me…. you, too. [That's just who I am.] Researching this was not easy, but it was important. A study published in 2019 in the journal BMC Nephrology, [Bio Med Central] explains why.

"Asian Americans (AA)s are projected to be the second fastest growing racial/ethnic group in the U.S and are projected to nearly double to 9.3% of the total population by 2060…. Currently, AAs represent 5.8% of the overall U.S. population … and there are approximately 20.4 million Asian adults and children living in the U.S. … Furthermore based on the 2016 U.S. Census, major Asian subgroups of people reported were Chinese (except Taiwanese) (4.9 million), Asian Indian (4.1 million), Filipino (3.9 million), Vietnamese (2.1 million), Korean (1.8 million), and Japanese (1.5 million)."

Well, what's the problem? Why isn't the eGFR accurate in these populations? I repeatedly read that it has to do with the lean muscle mass [Here we go again with muscle mass.] and eating little meat. I found little on the topic in medical journals and even less on websites re nephrology for lay people like you and me. However, PubMed did offer the following:

"Low muscle mass may cause considerable overestimation of single measurements of eGFRCr. Muscle wasting may cause spurious overestimation of repeatedly measured eGFRCr. Implementing muscle mass-independent markers for estimating renal function, like cystatin C as superior alternative to creatinine, is crucial to accurately assess renal function in settings of low muscle mass or muscle wasting."

The "Cr" at the end of eGFR means it was calculated using serum creatinine. Serum means blood.

And eating little meat? Whatever does that have to do with your eGFR? The National Kidney Foundation had that one covered in their Health Unlocked,

" ... meat (cooked) contains creatinine so when you eat meat your serum creatinine naturally increases. Serum creatinine is the serum marker whose value is usually used in eGFR calculations. And so your diet influences this eGFR measurement

Eat less (or no meat) and your serum creatinine will probably fall. Consequently, your eGFR would improve.

But that says nothing about your actual GFR (actual rate at which blood is being filtered). Your actual GFR is the true measure of your kidney performance, not an [sic] number which is being influenced by what you happen to be eating around that period of time.

Indeed, you might well find your eGFR is improving (because you've stopped eating meat) but your GFR (which usually isn't being tracked) is disimproving (because CKD is a progressive disease)."

All this talk of eGFR. Let's back track a little and talk about that. Way back in 2011, I defined the term in *What Is It and How Did I Get It? Early Stage Chronic Kidney Disease*, my very first CKD book:

"Glomerular filtration rate [if there is a lower case "e" before the term, it means estimated glomerular filtration rate] which determines both the stage of kidney disease and how well the kidneys are functioning."

Got it? Let's move on to the 24 Hour Urine Test, which is what my Asian reader told me her nephrologist uses to determine her GFR. How about a definition first? This is from Johns Hopkins Medicine:

"A 24-hour urine collection is a simple lab test that measures what's in your urine. The test is used to check kidney function. A 24-hour urine collection is done by collecting your urine in a special container over a full 24-hour period. The container must be kept cool until the urine is returned to the lab.

Urine is made up of water and dissolved chemicals, such as sodium and potassium. It also contains urea. This is made when protein breaks down. And it contains creatinine, which is formed from muscle breakdown. Normally, urine contains certain amounts of these waste products. It may be a sign of a certain disease or condition if these amounts are not within a normal range. Or if other substances are present."

Ah, now it makes sense. While creatinine is being tested, it is not the only thing being tested. Notice sodium, potassium, and urea are also being tested. Clever.

On another note entirely, are you aware of the number of CKD Facebook Groups there are? Quite a number are hosted by James Myers, better known as Uncle Jim. Why? In his words:

"I began to understand my role. I made a conscious choice. I wanted to help my fellow Kidney Patients. I wanted to use my loud voice to help others. I wanted to advocate for clinic mates who could not advocate for themselves. I did not like the way the dialysis clinics, the government and the care staff pushed around or neglected my fellow Kidney Patients. The last straw for me was when they began to push for the cutting of funds to dialysis patients and clinics. I looked around the room and I realized with my health and skill set, I was the only one who could help. It occurred to me that if I did not accept this responsibility, maybe no one else would."

Some of his groups and the ones he frequently posts on are:

CKD Patients Group

Dialysis & Kidney Disease

Encouraging Kidney Donation

Kidney Advocates

Kidney Cancer

Kidney Disease Ideas and Diet 1

Kidney Education

Kidney Help for You

Kidneys Stories 2 And Live Broadcasts With Uncle Jim

Kidney Transplant Success Stories (JM)

Kidney Writers

Kidneys and Diabetes

Kidneys and Insomnia

Kidneys and Medicare

Kidneys and Medications

Kidneys and Other Surgeries

Kidneys and Social Media

Kidneys and Studies

Kidneys and the Arts

Kidneys and the Coronavirus

Kidneys and Your Heart

Kidneys and Your Parathyroid

Kidneys and Vets

Living on Dialysis

Living with Chronic Kidney Disease (CKD)

Love Your Kidneys!!!

Pre-Emptive Kidney Transplants: Transplant Before Dialysis

Jim has over 95 groups, so it's obvious I haven't listed them all. That's due to a lack of space rather than favoritism. I like all his groups. Surely, there's something for you in one of these groups, so if you're on Facebook, peruse them and see which resonates with you.

10/31 Peeking into Peds

This has been a banner year for babies amongst my daughter's friends circle. It's too bad they're spread all over the country, but that's the way it is these days, isn't it? Anyway, one of these babies has been having a difficult time lately.

If you remember, I created **SlowItDownCKD** way back in 2011. I have never written about pediatric kidneys. But I was more than curious about how I might be able to help this young woman and her husband understand what her baby was going through. Therefore, welcome to my first blog concerning pediatric kidneys.

This baby boy's problems started with RSV. What's RSV? Let's allow the Centers for Disease Control and Prevention answer that question:

"Respiratory syncytial (sin-SISH-uhl) virus, or RSV, is a common respiratory virus that usually causes mild, cold-like symptoms. Most people recover in a week or two, but RSV can be serious, especially for infants and older adults. RSV is the most common cause of bronchiolitis (inflammation of the small airways in the lung) and pneumonia (infection of the lungs) in children younger than 1 year of age in the United States."

You're probably asking yourself what the lungs have to do with the kidneys at this point. An article in the Journal of Nephrology explains:

"A significant interaction between kidneys and lungs has been shown in physiological and pathological conditions. The two organs can both be targets of the same systemic disease (e.g., some vasculitides [Gail here: That means one of the disorders that inflame blood vessels to the point of destroying them.]). Moreover, loss of normal function of either of them can induce direct and indirect dysregulation of the other one."

The little tyke in question tested positive for a UTI. Take a look at what Johns Hopkins Medicine has to say about UTIs:

"A urinary tract infection is inflammation of part of the system that takes urine out of the body. It's caused by bacteria. The urinary tract includes the two kidneys. They remove liquid waste from the blood in the form of urine. Narrow tubes (ureters) carry urine from the kidneys to the bladder. Urine is stored in the bladder. When the bladder is emptied, the urine travels through a tube called the urethra and passes out of the body. Bacteria can infect any part of this system."

The baby's UTI was determined to be caused by E. coli. I have to admit I didn't know much about E. coli, so I turned to UpToDate, an easily understood medical site for professionals [and seemingly lay people], and not only found information about E. coli, but more about UTIs:

"In healthy children, most urinary tract infections (UTIs) are caused by Escherichia coli (E. coli) bacteria, which are normally found in stool. These bacteria can move from the anus to the urethra and into the bladder (and sometimes up into the kidney), causing infection.

Risk factors — Some children have a higher chance of developing a UTI. The following are some risk factors for UTI:

• Young age – Males younger than one year old and females younger than four years of age are at highest risk.

●Being uncircumcised – There is a four to 10 times higher risk of UTIs in uncircumcised males. Still, most uncircumcised males do not develop UTIs. ...

●Having a bladder catheter for a prolonged period of time.

- Having parts of the urinary tract that did not form correctly before birth.

- Having a bladder that does not work properly or constipation (bladder and bowel dysfunction [BBD]).

- Having one UTI slightly increases the chance of getting another UTI."

My daughter explained that her friend's little boy was uncircumcised and had both catheters [although not for extended periods] and UTIs before. Then she asked why the baby needed an ultrasound. As always, I told her I'd try to find out.

I not only found out, but discovered information about the other test this baby is taking:

"For a renal ultrasound, warm jelly is placed on the abdomen and back and a probe is moved over the surface of the skin. This produces a special kind of picture of the kidney and bladder. This picture shows the size of the kidneys and the bladder, and if there are any other problems such as previous scarring or swelling of the kidneys (hydronephrosis) or thickening of the bladder wall.

A voiding cystourethrogram is a test where a small tube called a catheter is inserted in the bladder. The bladder is filled with a dye and x-rays are taken. Once the bladder is full, the child is asked to urinate and x-rays are taken again. If the fluid with the dye is seen backing up the ureters to the kidneys, reflux is present."

Thank you to Dartmouth Health Children's for educating us about the renal ultrasound and the voiding cystourethrogram. Even though a three month old baby cannot urinate on demand [At least, I don't think he can.], the catheter will help obtain the urine.

Maybe a reminder of how urine works would be helpful here. This is from Cincinnati Children's Health Library:

"The kidneys filter the blood and make urine. Urine goes from the kidneys to the bladder through tubes called ureters. Where the ureters and the bladder join, there is a valve-like mechanism. This mechanism prevents the urine from backing up to the kidneys. As the bladder fills with urine, it sends a message to the brain. The brain then sends a message to the sphincter muscle to relax, while the bladder muscle squeezes, allowing the bladder to empty. This is called voiding or urination."

I think I skipped over 'reflux.' Let me check. Hmmm, I did. Okay, in this case reflux refers to the backing up of the urine. Well, it is a little more complex than that. Back to Cincinnati Children's Health Library for us:

"Vesicoureteral reflux (VUR) is a condition in which urine from the bladder is able to flow back up into the ureter and kidney. It is caused by a problem with the valve mechanism. Pressure from the urine filling the bladder should close the tunnel of the ureter. It should not allow urine to flow back up into the ureter. When the ureter enters the bladder at an unusual angle reflux can can [sic] occur. This can also happen when the length of the ureter that tunnels through the bladder wall is too short.

VUR becomes a problem when the urine in the bladder gets infected. The infected urine travels backward to the kidney. This can cause a kidney infection. Kidney infections lead to kidney damage."

Don't panic, mother of this babe. The reflux is graded from 1-5. In most cases of grades 1-3, the condition will correct itself as your baby matures. The baby will need to take antibiotics on a daily basis, however.

There's even more information available about urine reflex and how to treat it in babies, but this is a blog – not a book – so I'll have to stop now. To the mother of this little boy, I hope I've helped you understand a bit better.

11/7 Support Groups

I was speaking with my junior high school buddy, Joanne, the other morning. We don't speak that often, but our conversations do tend to be at least an hour. Yes, this is the same Joanne I wrote about in **Cancer Dancer.** She told me about the support groups she belongs to. No, not Facebook groups, but zoom groups that started out as in person support groups and what she gets from them.

I soon realized I've written pretty much only about the Facebook support groups. Well, it seems it's time to write about in person or zoom groups. Some of these support groups were solely in person until the pandemic began, at which time they began offering zoom meetings. Some offer both: in person and zoom meetings.

As someone who is a loner, I wanted to know what I could tell my readers about the benefits of support groups. MayoClinic to the rescue!

"Benefits of participating in a support group may include:

Feeling less lonely, isolated or judged

Reducing distress, depression, anxiety or fatigue

Talking openly and honestly about your feelings

Improving skills to cope with challenges

Staying motivated to manage chronic conditions or stick to treatment plans

Gaining a sense of empowerment, control or hope

Improving understanding of a disease and your own experience with it

Getting practical feedback about treatment options

Learning about health, economic or social resources"

They do have a lot to offer. My buddy also mentioned how good she felt when another member of the support group said something like, "As Joanne mentioned...." She felt like she helped someone. I can see that.

What about medical support groups? Are they different in any way? According to HelpGuide:

"When you're going through a challenging or traumatic time, family members and friends may sympathize, but they don't always know what to say or the best ways to help. Doctors and health professionals may sometimes offer minor emotional support, but their primary focus is always medical.

Support groups developed to join people together who are dealing with similar difficult circumstances. That may be coping with a specific medical condition, such as cancer or dementia, a mental health issue like depression, anxiety, bereavement, or addiction, for example, or caring for a family member or friend facing such a problem. Whatever issues you or a loved one are facing, though, the best medicine can

often be the voice of people who have walked in your shoes.

A support group offers a safe place where you can get information that's practical, constructive, and helpful. You'll have the benefit of encouragement, and you'll learn more about coping with your problems through shared experiences. Hearing from others facing similar challenges can also make you feel less alone in your troubles."

Hmmm, maybe we should look at the different kinds of zoom support groups now. By the way, I like the easily understood way Study.com delineated these:

"Member-only/Self-help/Peer Support Groups

Some support groups do not have a professionally trained leader. These are called member-only, self-help, or peer support groups. ... there is usually no professionally trained leader. These support groups are beneficial because members can tell their own stories, listen to other people's stories, and support and provide advice or strategies for one another. Sometimes members of these groups may feel more free to honestly share their thoughts than people in groups with a professionally trained facilitator, although this is not always the case.

Professionally Facilitated Support Groups

Professionally facilitated support groups are usually well-organized and have a leader who is professionally trained to help members deal with the group's core issues.... while the facilitator might or might not have personally experienced the issue at the core of the support group, they would be professionally trained and experienced in supporting people who are dealing with these issues. These support groups are beneficial because members can share their own experiences, listen to other people's experiences, provide support to one another, and receive professional advice and opinions about how to handle their particular issues. Members may also receive strategies to cope or improve from other group members. Some groups have leaders who have experienced the problem the group supports and who are professionally licensed to provide therapy to others.

Members of a support group work together to help one another and to receive support.

Online Support Groups

Online support groups may have a professionally trained leader, a leader who has experienced the issue, or no clear leader. These groups, like other support groups, can have any number of purposes.... The benefits could be the same as in-person support groups, such as providing an outlet to express feelings, the chance to help others, the opportunity to get advice and coping techniques, and an increase in positive feelings. A unique benefit of online support groups is that people who live anywhere can join as can people who have physical disabilities that limit their mobility.

Depending on the criteria involved in joining the online support group, one challenge could be making sure that members genuinely had the problem the support group was centered around. Online support groups that are not run effectively might be unmonitored, which could increase the chance of problems, rather than benefits, for members. However, overall, online support groups are effective tools for support."

I think we should spend a little time on where to find these support groups. Of special interest to us would be those for chronic kidney disease, dialysis, and/or transplant. A good place to start is the National Kidney Foundation. Their support group is asynchronous, meaning not all the members are online at the same time. You leave a comment or question, and other members answer when they can.

The AAKP, or American Association of Kidney Patients, offers a list of online support groups by state. At last count, there were 11 different groups. Some of them were further specialized as to transplant, men only, and end stage renal disease. Some even offered telephone entry to the group for those without computers.

RSNHope, the Renal Support Network, offers their own online support group. Many of the hospitals where you've been treated may also offer online support groups. Or you can ask your nephrologist if they can help you find one. Remember, if it's online, it doesn't have to be local.

What do you say we all give Joanne a big thank you for suggesting today's topic.

11/14 *It's Seasonal*

Now that I'm getting older [oh, all right, old], I see loads of specialists for my comorbidities. One of them, my rheumatologist, has mentioned several times that eGFR is lower in the summer and higher in the winter. I wondered why, but she'd already gone on to discussing my arthritis by the time I formulated my question. It seems like now is a good time to answer that question. Want to explore it with me?

A few reminders first. According to Medical News Today:

"A rheumatologist is an internal medicine doctor who specializes in diagnosing and treating inflammatory conditions that affect the joints, tendons, ligaments, bones, and muscles.

Rheumatologists diagnose and treat musculoskeletal conditions, but they do not perform surgery."

I started seeing her for osteoarthritis decades ago.

And eGFR? SelfCode, a site that is new to me which helps you decode your lab results, has that covered:

"Glomerular Filtration Rate (GFR) is the amount of blood filtered every minute by tiny filters in the kidneys called glomeruli. Although it may sound complicated, in essence, it measures how well your kidneys are working...."

Ready to explore the seasonal up and down of eGFR now? The first site that I could understand [Let's remember I'm not a doctor and never claimed to be one.] which explained the connection between eGFR lowering during the summer was from the European Renal Association.

"In general, our body has various ways of regulating the body temperature and releasing excess heat. The best-known method is through sweating. If the temperature control centre in our brain, known as the 'hypothalamus', detects that our comfort body temperature of 37 degrees [That's Celsius; it's 98.6 Fahrenheit.] exceeded, the sweat glands in the skin are stimulated to produce more. We consequently give off heat by 'evaporating' the sweat on the surface of the body. In addition, the body dilates our skin vessels. The heart pumps more warm blood into the dilated skin vessels, which also dissipates heat.

The increased sweating naturally leads to a loss of fluid and important body salts, the so-called electrolytes. The lack of fluid and the heat-induced widening of the vessels lead to a drop in blood pressure. The heart no longer pumps enough blood through the body and the kidneys," explains Professor Dr. Christoph Wanner, Head of Nephrology at the German University Hospital in Würzburg and President of the European Renal Association (ERA). 'If you don't compensate for this fluid loss, you become dehydrated. This can result in kidney failure. The risk to develop urinary stones and urinary tract infections is also bigger when the body is dehydrated.'"

Now this may look like it doesn't address the question, but remember we need to keep hydrated to keep the eGFR up. Increased sweating is a factor. Losing fluid and electrolytes is a factor. Widening of the vessels is a factor. A drop in blood pressure is a factor. The kidneys not receiving enough blood is a factor.

Well, it seems my rheumatologist is right about lower eGFR in the summer. Wait a minute. That means she's correct about a higher eGFR in the winter. Logically, if something is lower in some instances, it's higher in others. Medically, we can work this backwards.

If the kidney disease patient is not abundantly sweating, then they are not losing fluid and electrolytes. If they are not losing fluid and electrolytes, their blood vessels are not widening. If their blood vessels are not widening, their blood pressure is not dropping. If their blood pressure is not dropping, the kidneys are receiving enough blood. If the kidneys are receiving enough blood, your eGFR will be higher than it would be if none of this were the case. Voila! There we have a higher [than summer] eGFR in the winter.

I thought it was interesting that blood pressure is also usually lower during the summer. The Mayo Clinic has the information on this:

"Blood pressure can be affected in summer weather because of the body's attempts to radiate heat. High temperatures and high humidity can cause more blood flow to the skin. This causes the heart to beat faster while circulating twice as much blood per minute than on a normal day.

The greatest risks are when the temperature is above 70 degrees F and the humidity is more than 70%. The higher the humidity, the more moisture in the air.

Some people are at higher risk of being affected by humidity, including people over 50; those who are overweight; or those who have heart, lung or kidney conditions.

Heat and sweating also can lower the amount of fluid in the body, which can reduce blood volume and lead to dehydration. This can interfere with the body's ability to cool off and may create strain on the heart.

Other risk factors include:

- Adults with heart, lung and kidney problems
- Seniors who follow a low-salt or low-sodium diet

- People who have a circulatory disease or problems with circulation
- Adults who take diuretics, sedatives and blood pressure medication"

11/21 *Back to Peds*

For someone who never planned to write about pediatric kidney issues, here I am again writing about pediatric kidney issues. It seems the mothers of all those babies in my life I've mentioned before like to visit me. One of them was a bit upset during her visit, so – being me – I asked what was wrong.

Her answer was surprising. It seems her little one [I think he's about five months old] was born with urine reflux in both kidneys. I'd heard of reflux before, but urine reflex? She explained and I wondered why she wasn't more upset. She explained that, too. But, as usual, I'm getting ahead of myself.

Let's start with what it is. First of all, she used the term VUR before telling me it was urine reflux. Well, what's the 'V' stand for? Turns out the medical term for this condition is VUR or Vesicoureteral Reflux. Okay, so what's that? I turned to one of my old reliable sources for the answer, NIDDK, which is the National Institute of Diabetes and Digestive and Kidney Diseases.

"Vesicoureteral reflux (VUR) is a condition in which urine flows backward from the bladder to one or both ureters and sometimes to the kidneys. VUR is most common in infants and young children. Most children don't have long-term problems from VUR.

Normally, urine flows down the urinary tract, from the kidneys, through the ureters, to the bladder. With VUR, some urine will flow back up—or reflux—through one or both ureters and may reach the kidneys....

VUR can cause urinary tract infections (UTI) [Gail here: A UTI may be the signal to test for VUR.] and, less commonly, kidney damage. The two main types of VUR are primary VUR and secondary VUR. Most children have primary VUR."

Oh, then what's secondary VUR? Thank you to the Cleveland Clinic for the following information:

"Secondary VUR occurs when a blockage in the urinary tract causes an increase in pressure and pushes urine back up from the urethra into your child's bladder, ureters and even kidneys. The blockage could result from an abnormal fold of tissue in the urethra that keeps urine from flowing freely out of your child's bladder. Another cause of secondary VUR might be a problem with nerves that cannot stimulate the bladder to release urine. Children with secondary VUR often have bilateral reflux."

I asked the dad - since I felt I was leaving him out of the conversation - if the baby had bilateral reflux. Yes, he did. But then the dad explained that there are five grades of VUR. This is starting to get a bit complicated. I turned to The Urology Care Foundation for help in understanding this:

"Grade I: urine reflux into the ureter only

Grade II: urine reflux into the ureter and the renal pelvis (where the ureter meets the kidney), without distention (swelling with fluid, or hydronephrosis)

Grade III: reflux into the ureter and the renal pelvis, causing mild swelling

Grade IV: results in moderate swelling

Grade V: results in severe swelling and twisting of the ureter"

Let's say VUR is suspected. What now? Cedars-Sinai explained:

"Voiding cystourethrogram (VCUG). A VCUG is a type of X-ray that examines the urinary tract. The healthcare provider puts a thin, flexible tube (catheter) in the urethra. This tube drains urine from the bladder to the outside of the body. The provider fills the bladder with a liquid dye. X-ray images are taken as the bladder fills and empties. The images will show if there is any reverse flow of urine into the ureters and kidneys.

Renal ultrasound (sonography). This is a painless test that uses sound waves and a computer to create images of body tissues. During the test, a healthcare provider moves a device called a transducer over the belly in the kidney area. This sends a picture of the kidney to a video screen. The healthcare provider can see the size and shape of the kidney. He or she can also see a growth, kidney stone, cyst, or other problems."

Wait a minute. I'd forgotten that each of the parents had explained this to me at different times.

Of course, my primary concern was what do you do about VUR? Again, the parents of the baby had explained, but I wanted to give you a medical source, in addition, so I went to Mayo Clinic:

"UTIs require prompt treatment with antibiotics to keep the infection from moving to the kidneys. To prevent UTIs, doctors may also prescribe antibiotics at a lower dose than for treating an infection.

A child being treated with medication needs to be monitored for as long as he or she is taking antibiotics. This includes periodic physical exams and urine tests to detect breakthrough infections — UTIs that occur despite the antibiotic treatment — and occasional radiographic scans of the bladder and kidneys to determine if your child has outgrown vesicoureteral reflux.

Surgery

Surgery for vesicoureteral reflux repairs the defect in the valve between the bladder and each affected ureter. A defect in the valve keeps it from closing and preventing urine from flowing backward.

Methods of surgical repair include:

Open surgery. Performed using general anesthesia, this surgery requires an incision in the lower abdomen through which the surgeon repairs the problem. This type of surgery usually requires a few days' stay in the hospital, during which a catheter is kept in place to drain your child's bladder. Vesicoureteral reflux may persist in a small number of children, but it generally resolves on its own without need for further intervention.

Robotic-assisted laparoscopic surgery. Similar to open surgery, this procedure involves repairing the valve between the ureter and the bladder, but it's performed using small incisions. Advantages include smaller incisions and possibly less bladder spasms than open surgery.

But, preliminary findings suggest that robotic-assisted laparoscopic surgery may not have as high of a success rate as open surgery. The procedure was also associated with a longer operating time, but a shorter hospital stay.

Endoscopic surgery. In this procedure, the doctor inserts a lighted tube (cystoscope) through the urethra to see inside your child's bladder, and then injects a bulking agent around the opening of the affected ureter to try to strengthen the valve's ability to close properly.

This method is minimally invasive compared with open surgery and presents fewer risks, though it may not be as effective. This procedure also requires general anesthesia, but generally can be performed as outpatient surgery."

Don't miss the key word in today's blog: OUTGROWN. It is possible for babies to outgrow VUS.

11/28 *These are not the Lucky Kind*

We all know about the superstition that horseshoes are lucky. Some might even argue that this is fact, not a superstition. Today, I'll be writing about the unlucky kind of horseshoe. Some of you may know about this already; some may not. I didn't and was surprised by what I found.

First off, a definition of horseshoe kidneys [Surprise!] might be helpful. WebMD was pretty comprehensive in their definition:

"Horseshoe kidney, also called renal fusion, is a condition that starts before a child is born.

As a baby develops in the womb, their kidneys move into position just above the waist -- one on each side of the body. But sometimes that doesn't happen as it should. Instead, the kidneys fuse together at their base, forming a U or horseshoe shape. It usually happens between weeks 7 and 9 of the pregnancy.

The condition isn't common -- about 1 in 500 babies have it, boys more often than girls. And many kids won't have serious health issues because of it.

However, about one in three children with fused kidneys will also have a problem with their heart, blood vessels, nervous system, reproductive or urinary systems, digestive system, or bones. There's no cure for renal fusion, but your child's doctor can help them manage those conditions."

Oh, so we're back in pediatrics again. I'm glad I decided to write about pediatric kidney problems once my first grandson was born a little over three years ago. My daughter tells me she and her friends find my pediatric kidney blogs helpful. At least, that's what I think she said. Here's hoping every parent finds the pediatric kidney blogs helpful.

Back to the topic at hand... or kidney, rather. Of course, my next step was to find out what causes horseshoe kidney. Thanks are due to MedicalNewsToday for the following information:

"Doctors are not sure what causes horseshoe kidney, but certain factors seem to raise the risk.

People with certain chromosomal disorders have a higher chance of also having horseshoe kidney. These disorders include:

Edwards syndrome

Turner syndrome

Down syndrome

However, having horseshoe kidney does not necessarily mean a person has a chromosomal abnormality. Other factors that scientists associate with horseshoe kidney include:

alcohol consumption during pregnancy

glycemic control due to diabetes

exposure to certain drugs during pregnancy, such as thalidomide

Doctors no longer give thalidomide to pregnant people, but some people affected by the drug still survive today."

I reasoned that we all know what Down syndrome is, but not necessarily the other two syndromes. I turned to Symptoms and Treatments for explanations:

"Edwards syndrome is a chromosomal abnormality characterized by the presence of an extra copy of genetic material on the 18th chromosome, either in whole or in part. The additional chromosome usually occurs before conception. The effects of the extra copy vary greatly, depending on the extent of the extra copy, genetic history, and chance.

This disorder [Turner syndrome] also known as gonadal dysgenesis affects women whose X chromosome is missing or have other abnormalities with one of their sex chromosomes. Normal females have forty six chromosomes comprising two X chromosomes. When one has Turner syndrome, he or she has one X chromosome and if the two are present, one of them is usually abnormal."

I wondered if there were symptoms. Boston Children's Hospital answered that question:

"While each child may experience symptoms differently, the most common symptoms of horseshoe kidney include:

urinary tract infection: usually uncommon in children under 5 years and unlikely in boys at any age

kidney stones: if the stones remain in the kidney, your child may have no symptoms. If the stones pass through her urinary tract, she could experience the following symptoms:

flank (around the side, just above the waist) pain

restlessness

sweating

nausea and/or vomiting

blood in urine

changes in urinary frequency

chills

fever

cloudy urine

hydronephrosis: occurs when there is a urinary tract obstruction and the kidney(s) become enlarged and potentially damaged. Symptoms of hydronephrosis may include the following:

abdominal mass

poor weight gain

decreased urination

urinary tract infection

About one-third of children with horseshoe kidney have no symptoms."

How do you even know your baby has horseshoe kidneys? I suppose you could tell by the symptoms, but some babies don't have any symptoms. Children's National clarified the diagnostic procedure for horseshoe kidneys:

"The healthcare provider will ask about your child's symptoms and health history. He or she may also ask about your family's health history. He or she will give your child a physical exam. Your child may also have tests, such as:

Renal ultrasound (sonography). This is a painless test that uses sound waves and a computer to create images of body tissues. During the test, a healthcare provider moves a device called a transducer over the belly in the kidney area. This sends a picture of the kidney to a video screen. The healthcare provider can see the size and shape of the kidney. He or she can also see a growth, kidney stone, cyst or other problems.

Mag-3 diuretic renal scan. A diagnostic nuclear imaging technique that is conducted by injecting a radioactive fluid into the vein. The radioactive material is then carried to the kidneys where it gives off signals that can be picked up by cameras. Midway during the procedure a diuretic medication is given to speed up urine flow through the kidneys. This helps detect any area of blockage in the urinary tract.

Blood tests. These look at how well the kidneys are working.

Urine test. This test checks for chemicals in the urine and signs of infection."

Babies grow up. What happens to adults who have horseshoe kidneys? The article: Renal outcomes in adult patients with horseshoe kidney pulled no punches:

"Patients with HSK [horseshoe kidney] are at risk of ESRD [End Stage Renal Disease], which may be attributable to the high prevalence of complications. Accordingly, these patients should be regarded as having chronic kidney disease and require regular monitoring of both kidney function and potential complications."

12/5 *Oh, Those Dimples!*

Most often when you see a doctor, he or she will press your leg with one of his fingers, look at the indent made that quickly pops back to normal, and murmur, "Hmmm." That's what my rheumatologist did last time I saw her, only she didn't say, "Hmmm." She said, "Look at that, Gail." Uh-oh.

I looked… and saw the indent still there. I know what that meant: edema. My favorite dictionary since high school almost 50 years ago, Merriam-Webster, defines edema for us:

"an abnormal infiltration and excess accumulation of serous fluid in connective tissue or in a serous cavity

called also dropsy"

So that's what dropsy is. I'd always wondered.

Back to the matter at hand. What does edema have to do with chronic kidney disease – if anything.

Comprehensive Vascular Care, a practice in Michigan, offered some facts new to me:

"It's also linked to two other major diseases: 1 in 3 adults with diabetes and 1 in 5 adults with high blood pressure may also have kidney disease. All three conditions can lead to edema (swelling) in the legs."

I realized when I read this that my endocrinologist, primary care doctor, and nephrologist also always checked for edema. How did I not know the connection between their specialties and edema?

After having written the blog for over a decade, it occurs to me that you may not know, either. Let's find out together.

We know the simple test of pressing a finger into your leg to determine if edema is present. MedicineNet tells us there are other tests which may be used to figure out if you have edema:

"X-ray

Electrocardiogram (EKG)

Blood tests

Urinalysis (urine test)"

Let's say it is found that you have edema. Sure, it may be associated with your CKD, high blood pressure, or/and diabetes, but how?

"You probably know your kidneys help eliminate fluids from your body through urination. But, kidneys also filter fluids, removing excess waste products from your blood. If your kidneys don't work properly, fluid can get trapped in your body. Some waste products, such as sodium, can cause fluid to get trapped in your soft tissues and cause swelling under your skin.

Kidney disease can cause swelling — or edema — anywhere in the body, but it's most common in the feet, andkles [sic], and lower legs — all areas affected most by gravity. Some people also have swelling in their hands or face.

If there's a lot of swelling, you might notice that when you press the swollen skin with your finger, the area stays dimpled or 'pitted' even after you remove your finger. This is sometimes called pitting edema, and it's typically associated with more severe edema.

If your tissues continue to swell, this will put more pressure on your skin, and your skin may look shiny or taut in the affected areas. Your skin may also be more prone to cuts and sores because it's stretched out. Some people develop skin ulcers, which are deep sores that take a long time to heal."

Thanks to Houston Kidney Specialist Center for the above information.

 Specialists of Tulsa helped out here:

"Edema has many causes, some much more serious than others. It can result from standing or walking in excessive heat; sitting for prolonged periods; eating too much salt; getting sunburned; or being premenstrual or pregnant. More serious causes of edema include the following:

Lymph-node problems (particularly after a mastectomy)

Certain medications

Venous insufficiency

Congestive heart failure

Cirrhosis

Kidney disease

Chronic bronchitis or emphysema

Infection, injury or allergic reaction

A lack of protein in the diet can also cause edema"

While that's interesting, I still want to know what it is in the kidneys specifically that causes edema.

I found one answer on the Mayo Clinic's site:

"Nephrotic syndrome is a kidney disorder that causes your body to pass too much protein in your urine.

Nephrotic syndrome is usually caused by damage to the clusters of small blood vessels in your kidneys that filter waste and excess water from your blood. The condition causes swelling, particularly in your feet and ankles, and increases the risk of other health problems."

Johns Hopkins Medical had more of the detail I was looking for:

"Nephrotic syndrome results from damage to the kidneys' glomeruli. These are the tiny blood vessels that filter waste and excess water from the blood and send them to the bladder as urine.

Your glomeruli keep protein in the body. When they are damaged, protein leaks into the urine. Healthy kidneys allow less than 1 gram of protein to spill into the urine in a day. In nephrotic syndrome, the glomeruli let 3 grams or more of protein to leak into the urine during a 24-hour period.

Nephrotic syndrome may happen with other health problems, such as kidney disease caused by diabetes and immune disorders. It can also develop after damage from viral infections.

The cause of nephrotic syndrome is not always known."

So, what do we do about edema? According to National Health Service of the UK:

"You may be advised to reduce your daily salt and fluid intake, including fluids in food such as soups and yoghurts, to help reduce the swelling.

In some cases you may also be given diuretics (tablets to help you pee more), such as furosemide.

Side effects of diuretics can include dehydration and reduced levels of sodium and potassium in the blood."

12/12 *And So It Begins*

I was looking for some notes I'd made for today's blog and couldn't find them. Okay, so my office is being rearranged. After a few minutes of my kind of cursing [quite inventive, if I do say so myself], I accepted that I would just have to recreate them. Certainly not from memory since chemo brain and chronic kidney disease brain fog share the space in my brain. Yep, I was going to go back to the internet and research the topic all over again.

But I didn't. I stumbled upon some information that blew me away. I had never wondered about this, not even a little. What is it, you ask. Let me answer your question with a question: Have you ever wondered how your kidneys came to be? That's the information I stumbled upon, and it fascinated me. We'll probably have to rely on quite a few definitions, but it's still worth exploring. I'll place the definitions in brackets next to the word being defined. They were gathered from my own brain and various sources.

Duke Medical's site is what sparked my interest:

"Ascent of the kidneys

The kidneys initially form near the tail of the embryo.

Vascular buds from the kidneys grow toward and invade the common iliac arteries [the ones that carry blood to the lower extremities].

Growth of the embryo in length causes the kidneys to 'ascend' to their final position in the lumbar [the lower spine and the part of the back near it] region.

Rather than 'drag' their blood supply with them as they ascend, the kidneys send out new and slightly more cranial [Of or relating to the skull or cranium] branches and then induce the regression of the more caudal [a. Of, at, or near the tail or hind parts; posterior: the caudal fin of a fish. b. Situated beneath or on the underside; inferior.] branches.

This is a highly regimented procedure. What if something goes awry? What could happen then? Back to Duke Medical for some possible answers:

"**A. Duplication of the urinary tract**

Occurs when the ureteric bud [what eventually becomes the ureter] prematurely divides before penetrating the metanephric blastema [the other part of the embryo that becomes part of the kidney, usually the nephrons].

Results in either a double kidney and/or a duplicated ureter and renal pelvis ["The renal pelvis is a chamber where all the urine-forming ducts meet and further routes urine to the urinary bladder." Mansi Kohli.]

B. Renal-Coloboma syndrome

The Pax2 gene essential for metanephric mesenchyme [later to become nephrons, the filters in your mature kidneys] to differentiate into epithelial tubules ["Renal tubular epithelial cells are resident cells in the tubulointerstitium [connecting tissue between the cells in the tubules] that have been shown to play crucial roles in various acute and chronic kidney diseases." National Library of Medicine.] in response to inductive signals from ureteric bud, so mutations (even if HETEROZYGOUS [Two variations of a gene on the same locus of a chromosome]) can produce renal defects. Patients typically exhibit the following symptoms:

Renal hypoplasia [incomplete development] – due to reduced proliferation of the mesenchyme [tissue found in organisms while they develop] derived epithelia [body tissue that covers all surfaces of your body, inside and out] during development.

Vesicouretral Reflux [Urine flows backwards up into the kidneys and ureters from the bladder] – most likely due to improper connection of the ureter to the bladder or possibly due to inherent defects in epithelial cells of the mature ureter.

Colobomas (ventral fissures in iris, retina, and/or optic nerve) – due to failure of the optic fissure to fuse (expression of Pax2 is observed in ventral part of the optic cup and optic stalk).

C. Nephroblastoma (Wilms Tumor)

found in infants from 0-24 months of age

consists of blastemal [a mass of cells that is capable of becoming an organ or appendage], epithelial, and stromal [supporting tissue] cell types

associated with mutations in genes related to kidney development (PAX2, WT1, etc.)

essentially due to incomplete mesenchymal-to-epithelial transformation (i.e. the cells fail to fully differentiate and transform into cancerous cells).

D. Polycystic kidney disease

can arise due to a variety of factors:

loss of polarity: aberrant differentiation of tubule cells results in inappropriate location of Na/K [sodium/potassium] channels to the apical [apex] (rather than basal [base]) domain of the cells. Na+ is pumped apically, water follows resulting in dilation of tubule lumens [part of the nephrons, have no red blood cells].

Overproliferation: excessive growth of tubule epithelium can occlude the lumen causing blockage."

You have been incredible today reading a blog with all the definitions stuck in the descriptions. Thank you for bearing with me on that. I feel the mystery has been solved. I hope you do, too. Knowing how kidneys are formed, believe it or not, makes me feel more appreciative of them – even though I was already very appreciative of them.

12/19 *Bet You Never Heard of This Kind of Duplex*

I've been writing this blog for over a decade and am continually amazed that new topics keep coming up. There is so much to chronic kidney disease. Today's new topic is duplex kidneys. You read that correctly: not duplex housing units, but duplex kidneys.

Everyone know what duplex means? Haha, you're so clever. Indeed, we are turning to my favorite dictionary since college over 50 years ago. The Merriam-Webster Dictionary tells us it means,

"1a: having two principal elements or parts: DOUBLE, TWOFOLD

  b: having two complementary polynucleotide strands of DNA or of DNA and RNA

 2: allowing telecommunication in opposite directions simultaneously "

This is the adjective (describes a noun or pronoun) definition of the word. There's also a noun (person, place, thing, or idea) definition, and a verb (action word) definition. In our case, we need the adjective definition because we are describing the kidney. Specifically, we need definition 1a.

I know, I know, enough with the English lesson and on to the actual duplex kidney. A new source, Denver Urology Associates, explains duplex kidneys:

"Duplex kidney is the duplication of the ureter tube, which drains urine from the kidney to the bladder. The condition results in two tubes rather than the normal single ureter tube for each kidney.

Duplex kidney (also known as duplicated collection system) occurs in about 1 percent of children and usually requires no medical treatment. Medical concerns relate to obstruction of urine flow or urine flowing back into the kidney.

The function of the kidneys is to filter waste from the blood and convert it to urine to be dispelled from the body. The urine travels from the kidney to the bladder via the ureter tube. The bladder expels urine through the urethra tube, which emerges at the tip of the penis in boys and at the upper region of the vagina in girls.

In the duplex kidney condition, the kidney forms in two, duplicate parts with separate ureter tubes, as well as a separate blood supply. In about half of duplex kidney cases, both kidneys are affected with the duplicate ureter and blood supply.

These double ureter tubes may join together in a 'y' shape before they reach the bladder and combine their delivery of urine. Or in other instances, each duplicate ureter will drain into the bladder via its own attachment.

In either case, the result is the same — and generally the same as in a normal kidney with only one ureter."

Considering one of the babies in my daughter's social circle has been having kidney problems, I wondered what the symptoms of duplex kidneys are. I turned to the UK's Top Doctors for answers:

"Duplex kidneys and duplicated ureters that drain directly into the bladder rarely cause any symptoms.

However, if there is a complete second ureter, this often functions poorly and can be connected to a number of problems:

Urinary tract infections (UTIs) – problems in urine drainage make it easier for bacteria to enter the urine and travel to the bladder. Under certain conditions, infections can even spread up to the kidneys.

Ureterocele – the end of the ureter doesn't develop properly, causing urine to be obstructed and become backed up. The ureter begins to swell and balloon where it enters the bladder and the length of the tube may become swollen as more urine backs up along it.

Vesicoureteral reflux – urine is able to flow back through the ureter, sometimes even as far as the kidney. This may be because of an abnormal connection between the ureter and the bladder or as a result of a ureterocele.

Hydronephrosis – the ureter and kidney swell due to urine being backed up. This may be due an abnormal connection between the ureter and the bladder or as a result of a ureterocele, and can lead to kidney damage.

Ectopic ureter – the ureter does not connect to the bladder, instead being blocked or leaking into another part of the body. This can lead to vesicoureteral reflux, hydronephrosis, swelling, and incontinence."

Logically, the next question would be, "How are duplex kidneys diagnosed?" Children's Hospital in Colorado had the answer:

"A duplex kidney is most commonly diagnosed by using an ultrasound scan. This is a simple test that looks at the kidney and it is not painful. Sometimes it is necessary to do additional tests, which can include a voiding cystourethrogram (VCUG), where a catheter is placed into the bladder and X-rays are taken as the bladder is filled. Another test used to diagnose this condition is a renogram, where the function of the kidney is evaluated."

Now here's a surprise. This is what you do if your baby has a duplex kidney. Doctor of Internal Medicine, Anthony L. Komaroff, tells us,

"No treatment is needed. There is no harm to the kidney, though some people with duplex kidneys are more prone to urinary infections, reflux and blockages of the urinary tract."

I'm not a doctor, but that didn't sound right to me, so I looked at site after site to check on it. It turns out that while a duplex kidney may not need treatment, the problems they may cause do need treatment. That made more sense to me, especially as the baby I mentioned is being treated for vesicoureteral reflux. I have no idea if she has duplex kidneys, but it seems vesicoureteral reflux does need to be treated.

The Children's Hospital of Philadelphia put this into perspective for us:

"Duplex kidneys are a normal variant, meaning that they occur commonly enough in healthy children to be considered normal. They occur in 1 percent of the population, and most cause no medical problems and will require no treatment."

Oh, that means if the baby in question's vesicoureteral reflux was caused by duplex kidneys, she does NOT have chronic kidney disease. I know one mama who's going to be very happy when she reads today's blog.

12/26 *Another Connection I Hadn't Expected*

My husband may have pneumonia. Bear also vacillates between stage 2 and stage 3 chronic kidney disease. That, of course, got me to thinking. If he does have pneumonia, will it affect his CKD? Or did the CKD have something to do with his possibly developing pneumonia?

According to the National Heart, Lung, and Blood Institute,

"Pneumonia is an infection that affects one or both lungs. It causes the air sacs, or alveoli, of the lungs to fill up with fluid or pus. Bacteria, viruses, or fungi may cause pneumonia. Symptoms can range from mild to serious and may include a cough with or without mucus (a slimy substance), fever, chills, and trouble breathing. How serious your pneumonia is depends on your age, your overall health, and what caused your infection."

Well, he's older than I am and I'm 75, so if it is pneumonia, it could be serious. Bear is now on his second round of antibiotics, just in case it is bacterial. But wait a minute. We're trying to figure out if pneumonia and CKD are in some way connected, not if my husband is in any trouble here.

I took a chance and turned to the National Center for Biotechnology Information to find out since they often have helped me with information I needed.

"Infections are a major cause of morbidity and mortality in chronic kidney disease (CKD) patients. The relationship is mutual: not only infections are [sic] severe and difficult to manage in CKD, but infections also contribute to the progression of CKD and complicate its management…. Lower respiratory tract infections e.g. Pneumonia are common occurrences in CKD patients and are associated with increased risk of hospitalization, cardiovascular events and mortality…

CKD has long been considered an independent risk factor for pneumonia. The risk of pneumonia is up to 1.97 fold higher in CKD patients-1.4 times higher for outpatient pneumonia and even higher, i.e., 2.17 times for inpatient pneumonia compared with patients without CKD…."

By the way, the previous source is part of the National Library of Medicine which, in turn, is part of the National Institutes of Health. The first source is also part of the National Institutes of Health.

Let's look at this a little bit more closely. Most importantly, there is a connection between pneumonia and CKD.

Side note, I've had a lower respiratory infection. No one mentioned it was pneumonia. I wonder why? I'm certain I reported to the doctor that I had CKD. I always do. How did I not know about this? As I've mentioned before, it is amazing to me that after 11 years of blogging about CKD, I'm still learning about it.

Back to pneumonia. Let's see if we can root out something about the mechanism. I had to really dig for some answers. Several explanations were too medicalese for me; I just didn't understand them. Others talked only about acute kidney injury [AKI]. Yet others dealt more with only end stage kidney disease [ESRD]. I finally settled upon *American Journal of Physiology-Lung Cellular and Molecular Physiology* for this information:

"Although chronic kidney disease is most commonly accompanied by cardiovascular diseases and diabetes, there is clear cross talk between the lungs and kidneys pH balance, phosphate metabolism, and immune system regulation. Our present understanding of the exact underlying mechanisms that contribute to chronic kidney disease-related pulmonary disease is poor."

Oh my, Doctors Health Press informs us that unbalanced Ph can affect:

"Circulatory system….

Digestive system….

Urinary system….

Immune system….

Integumentary system….

Muscular system….

Nervous system….

Reproductive system….

Respiratory system….

Skeletal system…."

Did you notice the respiratory system? That includes the lungs.

Keeping in mind that phosphate helps filter waste from the kidneys, what does it have to do with the lungs and pneumonia? Here's Springer Link's explanation:

"For a long time, phosphate, the anion [Gail here: that's a negatively charged ion] that incorporates the element phosphorus, has been considered of minor relevance compared to its most studied parent calcium. However, the interest in phosphate metabolism has been remarkably increased in the last two decades. This has been mainly driven, among others, by two factors. The first one relates to the appreciation that hypophosphatemia (as well as hyperphosphatemia), has deleterious effects not only on bone but also on other organs and systems such as skeletal muscle, myocardium, the haematopoietic, respiratory and central nervous systems, in addition to sensory organs …. Further impetus has been fuelled by finding molecular mechanisms underlying congenital diseases characterized by hypo and hyperphosphatemia and discovery of drugs reversing the culprit mechanism."

Remember that hypo means low and hyper means high. Also, phosphatemia means of or about phosphate. I was hoping you would notice 'respiratory' included above.

As for the immune system, *Nature Views Immunology* states,

"The kidney has a central role in electrolyte homeostasis and the removal of toxins and so, when its function is compromised, normal immune effector cell function and intestinal microbial homeostasis are disturbed."

A different journal, *Nature Immunology,* offers the following:

"Of all the sites of the body subject to incursion by pathogens, the lungs represent the most challenging immunological dilemma for the host. Not only do the lungs represent the environment most frequently targeted by pathogens, their role as the organ of gas exchange makes their normal functioning critical for health and intolerant of collateral damage."

Uh-oh, so it is possible for pneumonia and CKD to not only be associated, but each can worsen the other. Not what I was hoping to find, but information that will be helpful in treating my husband's two illnesses.

Until next year,

Keep living your life!

Gail Rae-Garwood

Index

A
AAKP, See Association of American Kidney Patients.
Acute Tubular Necrosis, 69-73
Advocacy, 58-9, 97-100, 194-5
Association of American Kidney Patients,178-181, 213
ATN, See Acute Tubular Necrosis.

B
Black Nephrologists, see Nephrologists, Black.
Blood Glucose, 110, 114-7, 122-5, 150-1, 164
Blood Sugar, See Blood Glucose.

C
CGM, See Continuous Glucose Monitoring Device.
Coffee, 74-7
Continuous Glucose Monitoring Device, 166-9
Cortisol, 163-4
Covid, 23-6, 66-7, 156

D
Dialysate, 65-8, 141-3

Dialysis, 53-5, 65-8, 130-1, 135, 139, 141-3
Dried Urine Test for Comprehensive Hormones, 162-5
Duplex Kidneys, See Kidneys.
D.U.T.C.H., See Dried Urine Test for Comprehensive Hormones

E
Edema, 228-32
Exercise, 101, 103-4, 158-61, 176-7

F
Facebook Groups Administered by James Myers, 203-5
Fluids, 74-8, 229, See also Coffee, See also Water.

G
GFR, See Glomerular Filtration Rate.
Glomerular Filtration Rate, 197-203, 215-8
Revised Calculation, Asians, 201-3
Blacks, 197-200

Seasonal, 215-8

H
HMB, 174-7
Horseshoe Kidney, 223-7
HSK, See Horseshoe Kidney.
Hydroxymethylbutyrate, See HMB.

I
Immigrants, Undocumented, 52-5
Insulin, 30-3, 110-1, 118-9, 122-4, 151-2

J
Jail, see Prison.

K
Kidneys, 233-41
Duplex, 237-41
Origin of, 233-6
KIdneyX, 141-4

L
Lead, 105-9. See also Water.

M
Muscle Loss, See HMB.

N
Nails 145-9
Nephrologists, Black, 48-51

O
Origin of Kidneys. See Kidneys.

P
Pancreas, 30-1, 118-21, 150-2
Pets, 102-4
Phosphorous, 20-1, 63-4, 92, 129-31
Pizza, 170-3
Pneumonia, 242-6
Potassium, 19, 63, 85-6, 92, 126-8, 144, 203
Prison, 44-7
Protein, 19-20, 61-2, 90, 133-6, 171-7, 231

R
Recipes, 92-6
Renal Support Network, 88-91
RSN, See Renal Support Network.

S
Salt, 62, 137-40, 157
Skin, 34-8, 229-30
Sodium, See Salt.
Street Drugs, 39-43
Super Taster, 154-7
Support Groups, 210-14

T
Toastmasters, 56-9
Transplant, 23-4, 27-9, 46, 54-9, 118-21, 126, 135, 139

U
Urine Reflux, Pediatric, 206-9, 219-22
  Primary, 219-22
  Secondary, 220

V
Vesicoureteral Reflux, See VUR, See Vesicoureteral Reflux.

W
Water, 74-83, 105-9, See also Lead. See also Edema.

Gail Rae-Garwood

My Notes

Gail Rae-Garwood

Have you read my earlier chronic kidney disease books?

Available on Amazon.com and B&N.com

in both print and digital

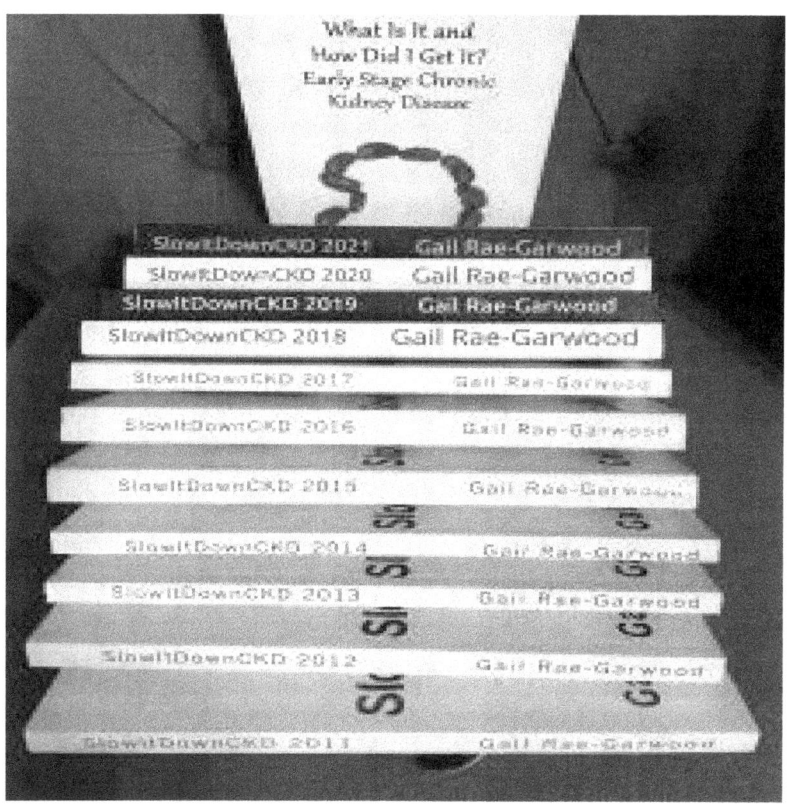

Gail Rae-Garwood

Follow the blog at https://gailraegarwood.wordpress.com

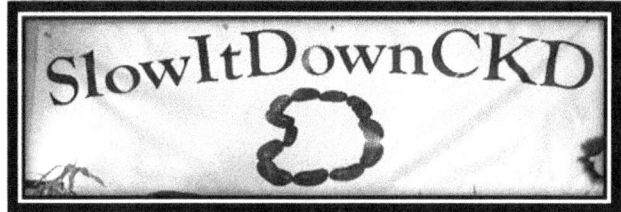

On Twitter, Pinterest, or Instagram, go to @SlowItDownCKD

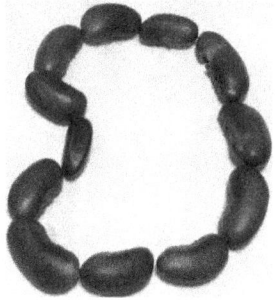

You can find me on LinkedIn as Gail Rae-Garwood

Then, there's the Facebook page at

https://www.facebook.com/SlowItDownCKD/

You can email me at SlowItDownCKD@gmail.com

Don't forget my website at gail-raegarwood.com

Gail Rae-Garwood

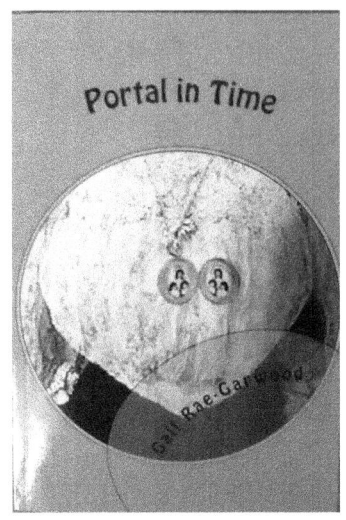

If you'd like to read a time travel romance (Portal in Time) or creative nonfiction based on others' experiences (Sort of Dark Places), I've written one of each. They're on Amazon.com.

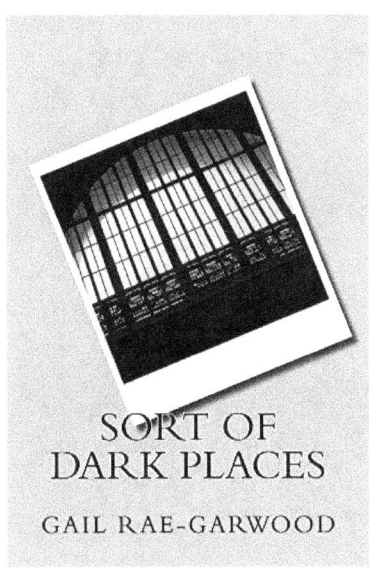

Then, there's my medical memoir, **Cancer Dancer**, which is also on Amazon.com. This book is about my dance with pancreatic cancer.

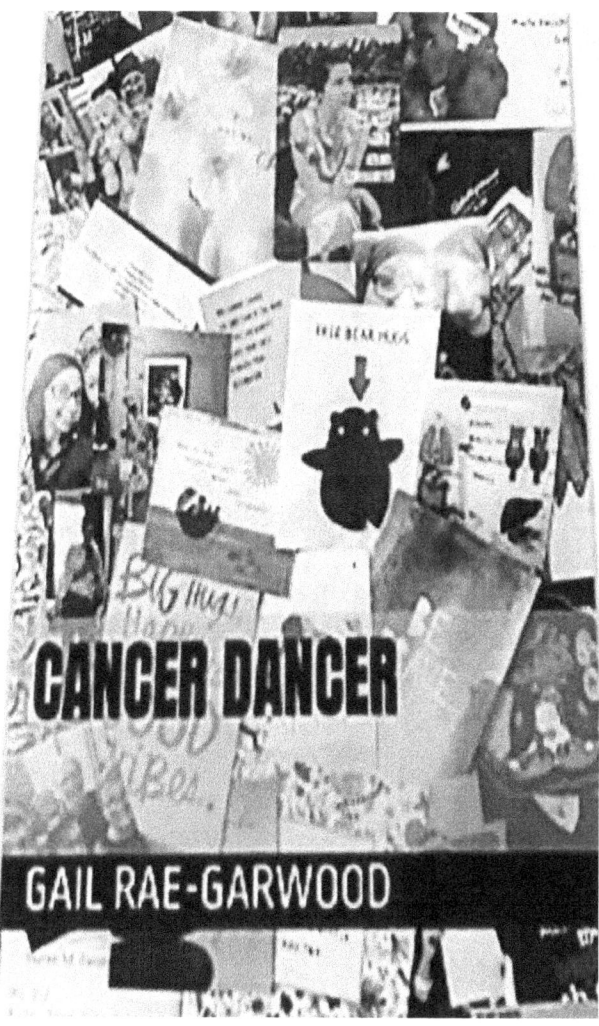

Gail Rae-Garwood

About the Author

While most of her work is non-fiction (how to, study guides, literary guides, and medical narrative), Gail also writes fiction; ***Portal in Time*** is a time travel romance. While writing it, she discovered that fiction is harder to write than non-fiction. Her quasi-comedy, ***Are You Kidding?*** is available on Kindle Vella.

Another of her non-fiction books is a compilation of short stories about ***Sort of Dark Places***, which is also the title. Her most recent book before this one is ***Cancer Dancer***, a memoir of Gail's journey with pancreatic cancer. All her books are available on Amazon.com.

Married, with two grown daughters, one son-in-law, and two grandsons she's crazy about, Gail lives in sunny, warm (to understate the weather) Arizona. She cohabitates with her husband, Bear, and their big, formerly white, fluffy dog, Shiloh. Gail retired from both college teaching and acting after a bit of soul searching about where her limited energy would be best spent. Having brain fog and chemo brain at the same time is no joke!

Gail Rae-Garwood

SlowItDownCKD 2022

Gail Rae-Garwood

www.ingramcontent.com/pod-product-compliance
Lightning Source LLC
Chambersburg PA
CBHW071352210526
45465CB00001B/62